# RESEARCHING
# PSYCHOTHERAPY
# AND COUNSELLING

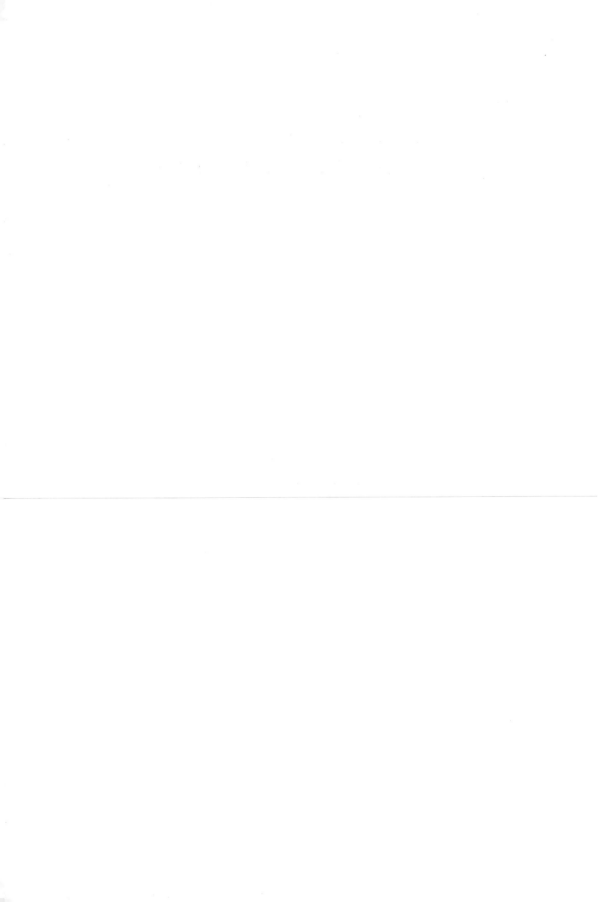

# RESEARCHING PSYCHOTHERAPY AND COUNSELLING

Rudi Dallos and Arlene Vetere

OPEN UNIVERSITY PRESS

Open University Press
McGraw-Hill Education
McGraw-Hill House
Shoppenhangers Road
Maidenhead
Berkshire
England
SL6 2QL

email: enquiries@openup.co.uk
world wide web: www.openup.co.uk

and Two Penn Plaza, New York, NY 10121-2289, USA

First published 2005

A catalogue record of this book is available from the British Library

ISBN–10   0335 21402 9 (pb)   0335 21403 7 (hb)
ISBN–13   978 0335 21402 0 (pb)   978 0335 21403 7 (hb)

Library of Congress Cataloguing-in-Publication Data
CIP data has been applied for

Typeset by RefineCatch Ltd, Bungay, Suffolk
Printed in the UK by Bell & Bain

# CONTENTS

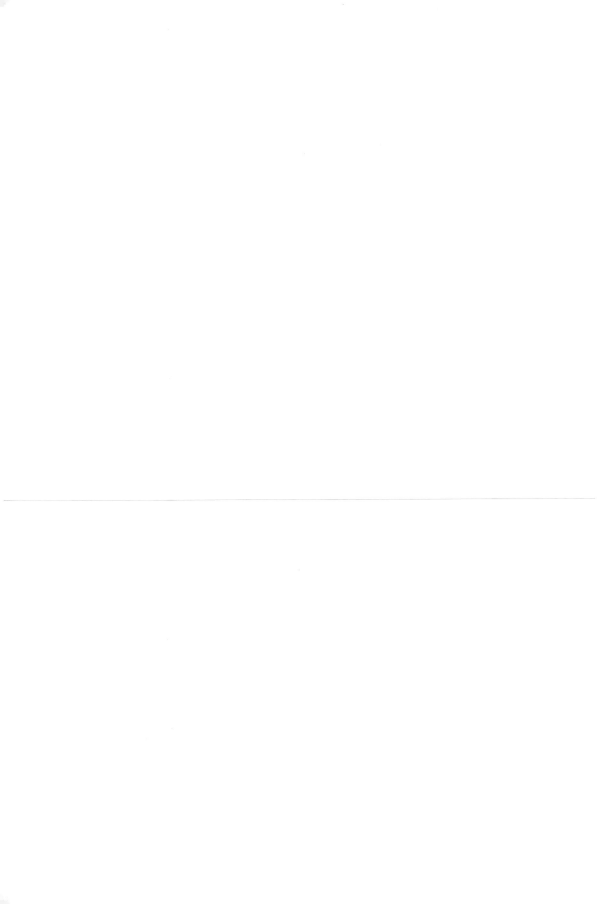

# PREFACE

## WHO IS THIS BOOK FOR?

Readers of this book may include practitioners who want to devote some time to explore a clinical observation, develop collaborative enquiry with user groups, explore the process of formulation and the relationship to change or question the relationship of policy to practice. They may also be practitioners who enrol on a higher research degree, or who undertake a further professional training in psychotherapy, and are required to complete a research project or dissertation. Readers may have been away from formal study for some time, may have little research experience or may lack confidence in how their previous research experience has stood the test of time.

This book is about researching the meaning of our clinical work and has been written with busy clinicians in mind. The aim of the book is to help clinicians develop do-able research designs that are based in clinical experience and that encourage reflective practice. Thus we aim to promote research design that is both collaborative and emancipatory in conception and practice for all participants.

In many ways, the book celebrates and legitimizes small-scale research as being within the reach of most practitioners and as making a strong and positive contribution to the development of theory and practice. We have paid attention to the ethics of accountability and have tried to stay close to the concerns and interests of practitioners.

Researching our own practice is the obvious starting point for the book. This could be about developing existing audit projects and imperatives into a reflective questioning of our own observations and practices; it could be about developing routine feedback from our clients into small-scale projects; it could be about joining with a few like minded colleagues into small clinical research teams and pooling skills, knowledge and resources into matters of common interest; or it could be about trainee counsellors and psychotherapists setting up pilot projects as part of their training requirements.

We draw heavily on clinical skills: observation, hypothesizing, interviewing and inferential thinking from single cases. At the heart of the book is the capable practitioner whose clinical skills are transferable to the research domain. Its aim is not to teach a course in research methods, as that has been done well by others for example (Barker *et al.*, 2002). Instead, we are trying to help busy clinicians maximize their existing skills and knowledge in the pursuit of systematic small-scale enquiry. For these reasons, the text moves from discussion of how-to-do-it guides to more in-depth and detailed discussion of the clinical and ethical aspects of the research process. In writing this book, we draw on our years of experience as teachers and supervisors of research, and on our recognition of our own needs as clinician researchers, as well as those of our colleagues who often approach us for consultation about how to get started in research. We have used Research Examples extensively throughout the text to illustrate do-able research projects in our public health and social care institutions.

*Rudi Dallos*
*Arlene Vetere*
*January 2005*

# 1     INTRODUCTION: RESEARCH IN

# PSYCHOTHERAPY AND COUNSELLING

## CHAPTER OVERVIEW

This chapter begins with an outline of the book in terms of four core themes that we argue should guide research into the structure and process of psychotherapy and counselling. These are:

- Collaborative and emancipatory research
- Reflective practice
- Experiential research: exploring the meaning and experience of our practice
- Do-able research design.

The chapter then examines the nature of the activity of psychotherapy and its aims to assist mental health. These are linked to questions of why we want to engage in research and what types of questions we may wish to ask: questions about evaluation, process, theory and the ethics of practice. The chapter concludes with a discussion of how these issues fundamentally connect with the concept of 'data' – what it is we are attempting to measure and how this starts to point towards designing research.

## AIMS AND ORIENTATIONS OF THE BOOK

The practices of psychotherapy and counselling have been increasingly subjected to the scrutiny of evaluation. Put very bluntly, the core questions have been in terms of whether psychotherapy and counselling are worth the time and expense involved. A critical focus has also been on whether, and in what ways, they are more or less effective than medical approaches. Since the drug companies invest large sums of money into research for new medications and advertising of their products, psychotherapy and counselling have needed to show not just that they can produce, but also that they can produce as cost effectively. Some of these pressures have led to the development of the 'evidence based' practice movement (Roth and Fonagy, 1996). This advocates that there should be clear research information regarding the effectiveness of different forms of psychotherapy and counselling for different types of psychological problems. Purchasers of therapy and counselling, such as managers in the NHS and individuals, can then choose, rather like medication, which variety is most suited to particular types of problems. This approach therefore forms an important context for the practice of psychotherapy and counselling.

In turn, this approach requires psychotherapists and counsellors to subject theory activities to appraisal through research. It requires us to gain research skills, varying from an understanding of research methods and findings to the abilities needed to conduct research ourselves. This book is an attempt to address this need. We acknowledge from the outset the imperatives of 'evidence based' practice and describe different approaches to evaluation and assessment of practice. However, we also explore some of the underlying assumptions of research into psychotherapy and counselling and, importantly, include in these questions what we mean by 'evidence' in such research.

The research process is often described as starting with some questions, refining these, finding a suitable methodology for exploring the questions, gathering some data, analysing it and writing up the results. This is a very straightforward view and often centres on questions of choosing a methodology and applying the correct statistical tests or analysis to get the results. For example, we may identify a question, such as how well a counselling service is working for young people who have been bereaved. We then want to work quickly because the answer is important and we want to know whether these distressed young people are being helped by what is being offered. We fully identify with the urgency that many clinicians may feel about the research process.

# CORE THEMES: ORIENTATIONS

While the last thing we want to achieve with this book is to squash enthusiasm, we do want to highlight some very important, in fact vital, features that need to form a part of the research process. The following overarching themes will form the framework for this book.

## Collaborative research: whose questions?

In the brief outline above, there is no mention of the involvement of the recipients of therapy and counselling. Traditionally, research has assumed a position of this being an activity that we 'experts' do to 'them' in therapy. Usually 'them' have been referred to as 'subjects', a term having some connotations beholding to 'royalty' via the scientist/researcher? We suggest that psychotherapy and counselling are intrinsically collaborative activities. Part of what therapists and clients are attempting to do is to understand each other, and importantly for therapists, to assist clients to be able to make sense of their own experiences. Research therefore needs to be consistent with the ethical and practical approach of psychotherapy, in that clients are active participants in research in terms of formulating the questions, methods, analysis and results, and dissemination of the research. Collaborative research also involves a variety of professionals, such as managers who purchase therapeutic services. In addition to taking account of their pragmatic needs, such as funding, they may also have a reservoir of experiences to draw on, for example, through involvement with clients and their families.

## Emancipatory research

This implies that research should be a considered an emancipatory activity. Many clients are disadvantaged and oppressed. For example, they may be poor, they may have been subject to abuse or torture, or they may have had a variety of discriminatory practices imposed on them, including unwanted treatments such as medication or electric shock treatment. Research into psychotherapy needs to take into account clients' experiences and circumstances and consider how research may assist in their empowerment. At the very least, we need to understand whether our preferred form of therapy is experienced by them as liberating or oppressive. For example, in many families that we work with we hear parents, especially mothers, describe how some sessions have left them feeling incompetent, irresponsible and blamed.

## The meaning and experience of psychotherapy and counselling

We suggest that in all research relating to human beings it is essential to consider the experiences of participants as well as the 'findings' of the research. In fact, we argue that the experiences and the findings are inextricably linked: experience is not simply an add-on. In psychotherapy this is perhaps even more crucial. People come for therapy usually because they are in pain, distressed, unhappy and sometimes on the edge of giving up on life or actively engaging in trying to end their lives. As clinicians we want and need to know not just if different therapies work but also how they work and how they are experienced by clients. What aspects start to make their lives seem more positive and worth living? What features enable them to feel they are competent and capable of taking charge of their lives and are worthwhile human beings?

## Reflective research

As in the practice of psychotherapy and counselling, the researcher needs to adopt a reflective position. This includes paying attention to what of their own experiences are driving their research aims and colouring the interpretation of the data. This applies not only to the analysis of qualitative data but also to quantitative data. In effect, the facts do not simply speak for themselves; research involves interpretation and we need to be sensitive to this. Incorporating clients into our research can help us to see our own assumptions, including ideas about issues of gender, power, inequality and ethnicity which are invariably relevant. In addition, in some forms of psychotherapy research, such as research into the process of psychotherapy, we need to reflect, as we do in our clinical practice, on the nature of our developing relationships with our research participants. In fact, if we are researching the process of our own therapy then such reflection is interwoven with our therapy.

## Do-able research

All research needs to be practicable, but we are suggesting that research into psychotherapy has to consider not only issues of time and cost but also a range of other important questions, such as the availability of clinical populations. For many busy clinicians it is not possible for them to engage in large-scale studies requiring large numbers of participants and external funding. However, related to the above themes this kind of research is not always what is of most value. Instead, it may be much more relevant to engage in research about their actual practice rather than, for example, studies that require them to work in quite different ways. Furthermore, clinicians may become disenfranchised from engaging in research unless it is relatively small scale and do-able within the constraints of their job. This may mean thinking about research, such as case studies, or small group designs that fit with their clinical practice.

Increasingly, such research has also come to be described as 'practice based' evidence and has figured strongly in the development of psychodynamic therapies and family therapies. Detailed description of clinical case work offered evidence that inspired many clinicians to review and revise their clinical practice. There is arguably a fine line between a good detailed case report and a piece of research. Hence an activity in which all clinicians engage can be seen as constituting the fundamentals of good research: clear description of the context of the work; descriptions of the participants; a clear and replicable account of the work that was carried out; evidence of its effectiveness by standardized measures; accounts from clients; and the clinician's observations. We are suggesting that research in psychotherapy need not, therefore, involve doing 'something else' – a burdensome add-on to our activity – but can involve doing what we already do and describing it in a clear and systematic manner.

These then are the key orientations and underlying themes that run through the book. We feel this offers a different orientation to many other books on research methods. We will review a variety of research approaches and outline details of methods. However, these orientations need to shape the start of our research process. They, therefore, require us to be more patient in our enthusiasm to find out if something works!

## KEY QUESTIONS ABOUT PSYCHOTHERAPY

### What is psychotherapy?

All forms of psychotherapy and counselling have as their aim positive outcomes for their clients. At first glance the aims appear quite straightforward and perhaps obvious: to help make people better. Conversely, we need to consider that the treatments do not actually make people worse. There are many examples in the history of medicine of treatments which were initially thought to be highly effective – such as administering insulin coma to people with a diagnosis of schizophrenia or performing colectomies (removal of the colon) on people with neurasthenia (now known as ME or chronic fatigue syndrome) – which turned out to be far from helpful (Wessley, 2001). When people are exhausted, distressed and depressed by their illness they want to believe that something can help. In medicine this has sometimes involved treatments that in retrospect may appear barbaric and abusive but at the time were seen as enlightened. Equally, we need to ask uncomfortable questions about psychotherapy and counselling in terms of whether they may have the opposite effect to what we all hope. There are parallels with medicine but there are also important points of separation. As a prelude to this book we need to consider some of the issues involved.

To start with, these revolve around the two issues of what counts as well-being, sometimes called 'mental health', and how we assess this. Social constructionist thinkers (Gergen, 1999) argue that social discourses are most pervasive and pernicious when they have a quality of being obvious, or 'common sense'. The term 'mental health' is a good example of the need to explore common-sense assumptions. Though much used as a concept, it is important to note from the outset that this term implies a medical idea of health in matters of the mind and emotions. It is much easier to define what it is to be healthy in terms of eradication of a physical disease than to define what constitutes 'healthy' thoughts or feelings. In fact, this activity has frequently been the domain not of psychotherapy but of religions, art and literature, governments and cultures, not to mention dictators and zealots!

## What is 'mental health'?

Perhaps this 'obviousness' is the case with the term mental health. Surely we all know what this is: isn't it obvious when someone is unhappy, distressed, freaked out, distraught, crazy, mentally ill . . .? As these words roll out though, we start to realize that actually they contain quite different implications. Some imply relatively temporary states of turmoil or distress that can be painful but actually are a normal feature of being alive. Others imply much more permanent states and possibly some serious fault in our 'hardware', such as brain chemistry, hereditary dispositions and so on. Perhaps the most pervasive and powerful definitions are about helping people to return to, or achieve a state of, mental health. Much of the research in psychotherapy and counselling has been directed to addressing the question of how effective the various approaches are in achieving this aim.

The most dominant approach to this question has involved the use of diagnostic systems, such as the DSM and ICD classifications (Diagnostic System Manual of the US Psychiatric Association; International Classification of Diseases). These adopt the approach of attempting to observe in careful detail and to classify forms of mental distress in a way similar to the ancient Greeks, who first developed systematic classificatory systems of plants and animals. Similarly, the DSM system classifies problems in a taxonomic system that consists of five axes: Axis 1 – clinical syndromes such as schizophrenic disorders, anxiety disorders and mood disorders; Axis 2 – developmental and personality disorders; Axis 3 – physical disorders and conditions; Axis 4 – severity of psycho-social stressors; and Axis 5 – global assessment of functioning. This system is based on behavioural and cognitive descriptions of problems rather than causal explanations, such as what people are doing and what kinds of thoughts and feelings they report or appear to be having.

Though ostensibly offering an objective the descriptive system, DSM has received a variety of criticism, not least that descriptions cannot be neutral and in fact privilege a behavioural–biological view of problems. There is also the question of how we come to know about these behaviours, thoughts and feelings. For example, it is not uncommon that referrals to mental health services come about as a result of other people, often family members making a decision that the behaviour of a relative is becoming unbearable. This typically becomes transformed into describing their behaviour as abnormal, odd, deviant or crazy. But different families, professionals and cultural groups have different ideas about what is normal and what is abnormal. When people eventually seek professional assistance, usually from a General Practitioner in the UK, they also have a variety of responses. Goldberg and Huxley (1992) have described this as pathways to mental health problems. Likewise, there has been a variety of research exploring how such processes of constructing problems and illness identities occurs (Kleinmann, 1988; Dallos et al., 1997).

Classificatory systems also assume a focus on the individual and some commonalities about the basis of problems. For example, the DSM and ICD appear to assume that the impact of any particular event in a person's life is mediated by some fundamental aspects of the person – their personality – not simply or predominantly by the event itself. As an example, depression is seen to represent some basic dysfunction in the way that a person processes events that have occurred in his or her life. In effect this implies that the person has or contains the problem(s), syndrome or disorder that can be classified and is then seen as the presenting problem.

A further issue is that DSM and similar diagnostic approaches draw on the medical model in that forms of mental distress are seen to be comparable to forms of physical illness. Careful and detailed observation, along with pragmatic experimentation, has produced some wondrous medical interventions. Sometimes these were fortuitous, as in the case of Edward Jenner's discovery of immunization, and at other times based on careful record keeping and detail, as in the case of Louis Pasteur's discovery of bacteria and his later observations that it was dirty operating conditions which had been the cause of much mortality following surgery. Both these discoveries have saved millions, if not billions, of lives. Such great gifts from medical science to humankind make it extremely tempting to assume that similar rewards will be produced in the domain of mental health. However, it is also worth noting that both the above medical approaches involve assisting the body's natural abilities to heal itself.

One of the cornerstones of the medical approach is that disease, infection and illness are destructive and dangerous states and success is achieved when we are able to return people to 'normal' as opposed to 'abnormal' functioning. But there are problems of applying this approach to matters of emotional distress. For example, what and where is the 'normal' place to which people should return? Even people who are in serious distress and emotional pain may want to feel more 'normal' in terms of reducing this distress, but once this has been relieved to some extent they may aspire to be individual, unique people with meaningful lives. Psychotherapy, therefore, involves a lot more than helping people to return to a 'normal' range on a diagnostic measure (Rustin, 2002).

In contrast, a number of other approaches classify symptoms, such as depression, as indications of other more profound processes. For example, psychodynamic approaches conceptualize problems in terms of unconscious processes, while systemic approaches conceptualize them in terms of a history and current pattern of interactions between key people in a client's life. Systemic approaches may go even further in rejecting the notion that a 'person' has a problem to a view that there is a particular interpersonal process that is problematic and leads to distress, for example, in all members of a family although they display this in different ways (Dallos and Draper, 2000; Vetere and Dallos, 2003).

However, DSM is the most widely used system to have been employed as a basis of research in psychotherapy, especially in terms of evaluations of effectiveness of psychotherapies and counselling. DSM is typically employed as the basis for the selection of 'patients' for studies that attempt to examine the effectiveness of treatments. Alternatively, and importantly in our view, research studies could be conducted that base their selection of participants not on DSM but, for example, on particular events that have been experienced, complexity of problems, patterns of family transactions or attachment styles. This underlines one of the problems with DSM, namely that it ignores what might be much more meaningful ways of grouping clients for inclusion in studies than just the behavioural manifestation of their problems. Furthermore, there has been a tendency to explore clients with conveniently distinct categories of problems, whereas in 'real life' clinical practice, as in the NHS in the UK, many, if not most, clients present with complex multiple problems, such as depression, drug dependency, self-harm and anxiety, possibly with different features more prevalent at different times.

In Chapter 5 we contend that rather than diagnosis, the process of psychological formulation of problems might be a better place to start research in psychotherapy. This might lead to studies that group clients, for example, in relation to how they regulate their emotional distress in terms of attachment styles, level of psychological mindedness or ability to process distressing material. Such groupings might be more psychologically meaningful and derived from theories of how problems evolve. However, even here we need to consider to what extent categorizations have the effect of excessively simplifying or reducing the complexity of the phenomenon we wish to study. Furthermore, all classifications can promote a sense that they are real rather than more or less helpful constructions. Additionally, we might even contemplate smaller-scale studies that explore individual experience in detail to offer a picture of the processes involved in problems and how these may shift in therapy.

## DATA AND MEASUREMENT

Alongside the above discussion runs the question of what constitutes data in psychotherapy research and counselling. In making decisions regarding who will be involved in a study, we need also to consider what we will gather in the form of data. Typically, there has been an assumption that this will include some measurement, some aspects that can be quantified. Broadly, we can distinguish between two types of evidence: quantitative and qualitative (see Table 1.1).

Quantitative approaches typically employ standardized measures, such as the BDI (Beck Depression Inventory, Beck, 1967) or GHQ (General Health Questionnaire, Goldberg, 1992), to assess how much change a group of clients has made during a course of therapy or over part of it. More

**Table 1.1** Types of data

| Qualitative | Quantitative |
|---|---|
| Idiographic | Nomothetic |
| Subjective | Objective |
| Internal states (thoughts, feelings, inner talk) | External states (behaviours, utterances) |

subjective approaches can also be employed, such as the use of ratings: for example, on a scale of 0 to 10, how much better does a person feel. It is even possible for clients to generate their own rating scales or measures so that change can be mapped in relation to their own beliefs of what they think are important areas in which they should change.

Qualitative measures are usually less concerned with amounts of change and more with the meanings that people give to what has gone on in therapy, how it has helped them to see things differently or supported their hopes that they will be able to manage. In systemic family therapy it might be that family members are able to see each other in different ways and feel more tolerant regarding each others' behaviours. More broadly, it might consist of data about a client feeling that life is more meaningful or even that they have a clearer sense that they are different but are happy to remain that way.

Second, our data may attempt to put together information about a group of people. For example, how people with particular types of problem respond to a particular type of psychotherapy. Alternatively, we may not be so interested in making such generalizations and produce instead an in-depth account of the responses of an individual client or a number of clients. For example, we might attempt to follow in detail how a person progresses through therapy. The data may also differ in the extent to which they are based on subjective measures. For example, they may be generated internally by a client or group of clients about their experience. This may constitute qualitative or quantitative data. It is worth noting that many so-called objective measures, such as inventories, require clients to make subjective ratings of how they feel. Questions, such as how depressed you feel (BDI II), require the person to make an observation of their own internal states and behaviour and compare it to some idea of what is normal or abnormal to them. Objective measures may be attempts, for example, to employ standardized observations, such as counts of the number of times a person engages in certain activities. The status of objectivity requires that the observations made can be verified by others.

Though related, the distinction between internal states and external states draws attention to the fact that people can make subjective estimates of external events, such as how well they think their family is functioning or how they are getting on with their therapist. In contrast, data about internal states relate to thoughts and feelings. So a client may report that his or her thoughts have been more hopeful about the future and that he/she has been feeling happier, less anxious and so on. Language can be seen in both aspects here: as external actions, for example, to whom is it directed, how much, what effects it seems to have on others; and as internal, for example, in how a client talks to him or herself. Many clients, for example, describe that their internal talk is extremely self-critical and negative. Significant therapeutic change may be associated with both the quantity and quality of a person's internal conversation.

Internal data can be conceptualized further, as they are in psychodynamic theories, as not easily amenable to either the client or the therapist, for example, unconscious processes and reactions. The therapist may infer internal states of which the client may not be aware, and in fact change may be seen as having occurred through shifts in these which requires interpretation by the therapist. This means that the data are subjective, not just in terms of the client's perspective but also in terms of the therapist forming subjective impressions about the client's experiences. This relates to the issue of the therapist's use of self and concepts such as transference and counter-transference. More broadly, it connects with the notion of data as hermeneutic and involving the researcher or therapist becoming immersed with the experience. Consequently, the nature of the relationship between the client and the therapist influences the data about the client and the meanings that are given to it.

We will return to some of these issues in subsequent chapters. In particular, in Chapter 5 we raise the question of the starting point for research in psychotherapy; in our view, it needs to be much broader than diagnosis and what DSM can offer. Instead, we want to suggest that a good starting point is the formulation that we hold about the nature of the problems we are exploring. For example, if we see the problems as due to difficult ongoing family dynamics, our research data need to be about such processes. If we see the problems in terms of unresolved impacts of a childhood trauma, we will want to collect data on whether the person is more or less able to process these experiences. Measures need to be chosen that are meaningful to the conceptualization that we hold about the problems and that are meaningful to clients.

Issues of power are involved in such choices. Psychotherapists have the status endowed by their professional qualifications, respect for their skills and power to involve other professionals in the lives of clients, coupled with the fact that clients are likely to be distressed and emotionally vulnerable. This means that we have to be careful to take time and be sensitive in inviting their collaboration and in working with them to produce preliminary formulations about their difficulties that are meaningful and respectful of their vulnerabilities. For example, it may not be satisfactory for us as clinicians to see shifts on an inventory as adequate data if a client still clearly sees their life as largely meaningless.

Let us now move on to consider what kind of questions we want to ask about psychotherapy. And why do we want to ask the questions?

## WHY DO WE WANT TO DO RESEARCH?

### What is our relationship to research?

There are many reasons why we might want to do research. Obviously it might be part of a professional training or part of our job description. What we are interested to explore here though are the many motivations and intentions that interweave in the complexity of our relationship to research. For example, what are the questions that we never ask? These might be questions that psychotherapists do not think to ask because they rest on taken-for-granted assumptions. Alternatively, we might want to do research to promote our brand of psychotherapy or to generalize our discovery of an adaptation to method. We may not choose to rely on 'author claims' to the helpfulness of our methods and approaches. We may wish to look at how different approaches to psychotherapy sit alongside other world views, and how we might do research across subcultural and cultural borders. Thus we might want to move beyond fashion and prejudice in psychotherapy.

Importantly, we would all wish to avoid potentially abusive methods and the risk that we might make people worse with our psychotherapies. Thus research could not only help to tackle questions of abusive practice but could also help to make a contribution to improved quality of life. Such honest hopes underpin many of the questions we ask as practitioners. We want to promote the asking of those questions in a research setting. Some critical problems stare us in the face, for example, developing services for people who are thought to have intractable problems, such as people with a psychiatric diagnosis of personality disorder. In Glenys Parry's (2001) preface to the Department of Health's *Evidence Based Clinical Practice Guidelines*, she concludes with her observation that nowhere is the gap between research and practice wider than in the field of psychotherapy. This is a challenge to us all.

We take the view that researchers should dare to question fundamental certainties and dominant fashions in psychotherapy practice, just as we expect practitioners to quest after the 'difference that makes a difference' (to paraphrase Bateson, 1972). It is for us a potentially subversive process. Research does need to have the power to shock, to say unpalatable things, to surprise us. Equally, we think we need research to establish our practice base, for without this confidence we are unlikely to ask difficult questions. If our wider cultural context of consumerism and complaint influences us as psychotherapists in any way, how would we know, and would it lead us to follow fashion and throw away tried and tested ideas? How can we maintain a position of scepticism and not be overcome by the emperor's new clothes? What are the influences that shape the questions that we start to ask? This book suggests ways of getting started as a researcher:

- Why do we want to do research into psychotherapy?
- What is our relationship to research?
- What is research?

## What is research?

Research is typically equated with the 'scientific method'. This is widely regarded as an approach to rigorous and systematic investigation that employs the process of hypothesis testing. We can note a number of concepts such as 'rigour' and 'systematic' that are included and privileged in this definition. Neither of these orientations are exclusive to science. For example, an artist can work in a systematic and rigorous way, taking great care and effort to produce exactly what they want. Furthermore, the definition by implication may serve to exclude activities, such as creativity, imagination and spontaneity. Typically, it is assumed that a deductive process is involved whereby hypotheses are derived from theory and tested, using methods of investigation and experimentation. Testing and retesting allow the development and revision of existing theory, and sometimes the abandonment of theory in favour of other explanations.

The scientific method of research can be seen as having provided huge benefits to the development of the physical sciences and technology. Interestingly though, Kuhn (1970) and others have argued that the process of research is not a straightforward, dogged accumulation of evidence, but may be seen as occurring through 'paradigm shifts'. These involve 'leaps of the imagination' or new and innovative ways of understanding the world and the evidence that is available. Some of these 'leaps' have been described as occurring in dreams or visions rather than simply as a dogged accumulation of evidence. For example, in physics, relativity theory was a paradigm shift from Newtonian physics.

This combination of systematic and sceptical thinking, with an interest in the recursive relationship between practice and evidence, is the hallmark of the psychotherapy researcher. In many ways this is also the hallmark of the psychotherapy practitioner. If research activity is going to become part and parcel of our activity as practitioners, there are a number of substantive issues that we need to consider. We highlight some of these below and expand on them throughout the book.

## Research questions and aims

- Are we interested in considering the effectiveness of psychotherapy and/ or the process of how change occurs?
- What is the population we wish to study? How are they to be defined: by symptoms, types of services they are receiving and so on?
- Use of self: what are our own interests, prejudices and backgrounds that shape the questions we may be wanting to ask?

## Participants

- What are our participants' motivations for engaging in a study that, for example, compares different treatments and randomly assigns them to a treatment?
- How do we set about researching some client groups who are typically difficult to engage in therapeutic work? (It is often convenient to employ clients who volunteer and are more willing to engage in research.)

## Choice of methods

- When to choose quantitative or qualitative research methods: how can quantitative research findings from group comparison studies (randomized control trials) help me when I see Mrs Smith?
- When to use participant observation or in-depth interviewing to hone our research question and/or develop our understanding?
- How do we examine the process of psychotherapy theory: for example, participant observation or the use of various forms of prompting to assist a client's recall and re-experience of the sessions?

*Value of research*

- The clinical relevance of our research: for example, do the results of psychotherapy outcome studies generalize to our working contexts – in the NHS, Social Services, education and private practice – beyond telling us that, generally speaking, these methods are helpful to people?
- How do we generalize findings from highly structured research settings – *efficacy*? How useful are therapies in the heat of complex local clinical practice – *effectiveness*?
- What is the value of local, small-scale, audit and/or qualitative studies to psychotherapy practice?
- The findings of the psychotherapy process studies and outcome studies: are we developing research questions that link an analysis of what happens in therapy sessions to outcome?

## SOME POINTERS FOR RESEARCH DESIGN

We conclude this chapter by offering some general pointers for thinking of research design and your approach to the literature review, and by way of introduction to Chapter 2, which develops our ideas for honing the research question. When approaching and choosing our research design, we need to question ourselves in five domains: our reasons for wanting to do the research; the social context in which we conduct the research; what it is we want to know and can know; how we can know it; and how we can trust our findings.

We have found the work of Colin Robson (2002) and James Maxwell (1996) helpful in our thinking about these points. We deal with each point in turn below.

 1 *Social value a utility*. In many ways this is the answer to the question 'so what?', or when your best friend asks, 'What was the point of doing the research?' What is your aim in doing this research and what questions flow from this aim? What is the social utility of the research and will it add anything to knowledge and practice (including training and supervision practice) in the field?

 2 *Social content*. This informs the conceptual development of the research question and includes pre-existing research and pilot work, clinical hypotheses and theory, as well as your clinical experience and personal experience. The social context in which you live and work will shape the direction of your thinking, including what we consider researchable at any time. Research supervision is crucial to helping us understand and deconstruct these wider, subtle and sometimes unseen processes at play in our thinking. Our awareness and understanding of these issues will shape the direction of our literature review and the support we can offer to our research question. Thus the research question will be seen to arise naturally out of the existing literature.

 3 *What is it that we want to know?* Our research aims will drive our research questions. These need to be feasible in terms of what we can know and the resources we can draw on. There may be more than one research

question and the reader of your research needs to know how they are connected. It is helpful to think about what we do not know and how that informs the way in which we frame our questions.

4 *How we attempt to understand and find out what we want to know.* We believe that the research question should drive the methods of data collection and data analysis we adopt. Our sampling strategy needs to include our choice of research site and methods of sampling. Our ethical and reflexive relationship with both the bodies of knowledge and questions we ask, on the one hand, and with the people who participate in our research, on the other hand, should be considered here.

5 *Trustworthiness of our findings.* To what extent can we relate our findings to pre-existing research and theory? How does our research sit within the field of enquiry more generally? On what basis should our readers pay attention to our findings and connect them to their fields of practice? Are we using our findings to support hypotheses? Do we pay attention to non-confirmatory findings? With hindsight, what might we have done differently?

## KEY REFERENCES

American Psychiatric Association (1994) *Diagnostic and Statistical Manual of Mental Disorders*, 4th edn. Washington, DC: American Psychiatric Association.

Dallos, R. and Draper, R. (2005) *An Introduction to Family Therapy*. 2nd edn. Buckingham: Open University Press.

Flick, U. (2002) *An Introduction to Qualitative Research*, 2nd edn. London: Sage.

Goldberg, D. and Huxley, P. (1992) *Common Mental Disorders*. London: Routledge.

Gomm, R., Hammersley, M. and Foster, P. (2000) *Case Study Method*. London: Sage.

Kuhn, T. (1970) *The Structure of Scientific Revolutions*. Chicago: University of Chicago Press.

Leff, J., Vearnals, S., Brevin, C. R., Wolff, G., Alexander, B., Asen, K., Dayson, D., Jones, E., Chisholm, D. and Everitt, B. (2000) The London Depression Intervention Trial. Randomised control trial of antidepressants vs couple therapy in the treatment and maintenance of people with depression living with a critical partner: clinical outcome and costs, *British Journal of Psychiatry*, 177: 95–100.

Mason, J. (2002) *Qualitative Researching*, 2nd edn. London: Sage.

Maxwell, J. (1996) *Qualitative Research Design: An Interactive Approach*. Thousand Oaks, CA: Sage.

Neuendorf, K. A. (2002) *The Content Analysis Guidebook*. London: Sage.

Robson, C. (2002) *Real World Research*, 2nd edn. Oxford: Blackwell.

Rustin, M. (2002) Research, evidence and psychotherapy, in C. Mace, S. Morley and B. Roberts (eds) *Evidence in the Psychological Therapies*. Hove: Brunner-Routledge.

Salmon, P. (2003) How do we recognise good research? *The Psychologist*, 16: 24–7.

Vetere, A. and Dallos, R. (2003) *Working Systemically with Families: Formulations, Interventions and Evaluations*. London: Karnac.

Wessley, S. (2002) Randomised control trials, in C. Mace, S. Morley and B. Roberts (eds) *Evidence in the Psychological Therapies*. Hove: Brunner-Routledge.

**2**

# GETTING STARTED: GENERATING AND

# REFINING RESEARCH QUESTIONS

## CHAPTER OVERVIEW

This chapter describes some of the features of starting research into psycho-therapy. It outlines three main types of research – evaluation, process and theory building research – and goes on to look at how these all connect with the key strands outlined in Chapter 1: collaborative research; a focus on meaning and experience; and research which is do-able. The chapter emphasizes the need to include clients in the planning of research and to adopt a reflective position in terms of the researcher's own interests and prejudices. It considers how the research may be used by the reader in addressing the important question of generalizability of the findings and outlines how the practicalities – the do-able features of research – also shape the research questions and aims. It concludes by offering pointers to conducting the literature review process that runs alongside the development of the research questions.

## GENERATING RESEARCH QUESTIONS

Research is a process that extends and develops over time. The initial stage usually starts with some questions or curiosity about a topic or issue. The traditional view in the social sciences is that research starts with some initial questions which are gradually sharpened so they can be stated in a testable form. These are referred to as the research *hypotheses* which can then be explored and tested. Importantly, it is argued that we can never confirm hypotheses, only disconfirm them. This means that we can find evidence to support our hypotheses but there may always be another situation, context or variation wherein they may be false. We can never explore the whole universe. However, we can disprove a hypothesis since if it is not proven in one situation it means that it is not universally true.

This is the traditional view of 'science' derived from the natural sciences (Popper, 1934/1959). However, in practice, research and its development is much muddier than this. Like other forms of creative process there may be several strands of thinking, interest, pressures and demands that shape the research. We might be content, for example, that a treatment is usually effective with a particular type of problem even if that is not always the case. This is a statistical position whereby, unlike in the physical sciences, we may be more prepared to accept some uncertainty. In some cases there might be demands as part of organizational imperatives to prove the effectiveness of a therapy in order to justify funding for a service. Alternatively, we might be inspired more by curiosity in trying out a method, for example, to see what a semi-structured interview might reveal about how people experience a course of cognitive behaviour therapy (CBT). As for most creative activities, motivation and inspiration are central concepts. The research ideas need to be of interest in order to inspire the energy and commitment to carry out the research and for the results to be of value.

So whatever inspires us may initially be varied, complex, hazy and even contradictory. However, we eventually need to move towards a clarification of our ideas and interests into questions that can be investigated. This process of clarifying and focusing our ideas is not an easy or comfortable one. It is sprinkled with confusions, impasses and, at times, a sense of despair. But let us make a start. Our suggestion is that the questions regarding psychotherapy and counselling can be seen to fall broadly within three categories: evaluation, process, and theoretical underpinnings of psychotherapy.

## Questions of evaluation

This might include the following kinds of questions:

- What is the best treatment for people with diagnoses of personality disorders?
- Are narrative counselling therapies effective?
- Do brief therapy approaches only produce superficial changes leading to later relapse?
- How does CBT compare with systemic couples therapy and drug therapy for severe depression?

## Questions about the process of psychotherapy

This might include the following kinds of questions:

- What is the impact of the use of reflecting teams in family therapy (Andersen, 1987)?
- How do people experience the use of sequential diagrams in cognitive analytic therapy (Ryle, 1990)?
- What is the influence of the therapeutic alliance in counselling and psychotherapy?
- How do understandings of problems and of oneself change in the process of therapy?
- How do understandings about relationships and their relevance to the problems change during therapy?

## Questions about theoretical underpinnings of psychotherapy

This might include the following kinds of questions:

- What are the attachment dynamics in families with a member with a diagnosis of anorexia nervosa?
- What are the core schemas in people struggling with addictive disorders?

We are not offering these as exemplars so much as the sort of initial questions that might be rattling around in our minds as a precursor to research. We want to suggest that from this point onwards we are actively involved in 'research'. Research, in other words, is not simply or predominantly about 'obtaining' our participants, devising questionnaires and running statistics packages to analyse the results, but initially can be seen as a sort of mind experiment or development of clinical thinking. We have to use our imagination to anticipate and visualize what various consequences might be according to how we try to approach and answer our question. This initial process is summarized in Fig. 2.1.

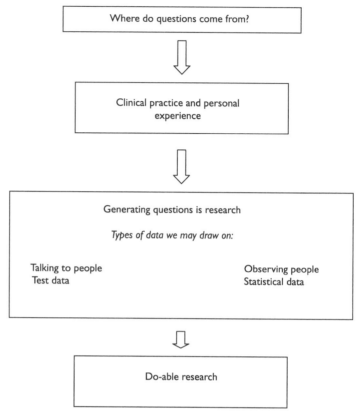

**Figure 2.1**   Generating research questions

## A REFLECTIVE AND EXPERIENTIAL APPROACH

### Deconstructing and reconstructing our research questions

One of the most fascinating but also, at times, most frightening and frustrating aspects of research is the process of critically appraising our research questions. This can sometimes feel like a form of self-critical rumination. Sometimes it seems that as soon as a good idea has popped into our head we have to take on the role of a grumpy critical research supervisor who finds all the flaws in our ideas. Importantly, these flaws may not only be *methodological* but also *conceptual*. Questions may arise from our clinical and personal experience, our observations and from available literature and data. We may also engage in some pre-pilot or pilot work as a prelude. We will outline these aspects in more detail, but before we do so it is important to bear in mind that this preliminary work can be very important and involves a mixture of active, critical and reflective thinking, along with a mixture of observation, talking to people and reading.

## Use of self

To start with, research questions inevitably arise from a personal position. This may be our clinical experience, personal experience, reading of the literatures and/or questions inspired by other colleagues. In taking a subjective approach, a researcher can explore his or her assumptions, expectations and biases, and at the same time look at how these are constructed within the wider social reality which we share with our participants and fellow clinicians and researchers (Rodriguez and Ryave, 2002). An obvious initial question here, for example, might be about gender and to think about what questions might interest a male as opposed to a female researcher. In the context of research into psychotherapy with eating disorders, for example, this might be extremely important. A pertinent social reality is that a far greater proportion of women seem to suffer with this condition (10:1) and a vastly greater proportion have engaged in dieting and are far more concerned about their body weight and shape than men (Fairburn and Brownell, 2002). Hence it is likely to be very important for the researcher to reflect on his or her own assumptions and experiences and how these are shaped by the dominant cultural values in all stages of the research. Initially, we might want to include some reflective questions, such as:

- What questions am I interested in?
- Why am I interested in these questions?
- How are my interests shaped by my own clinical and personal experience?
- In what ways are my questions shaped by wider culturally shared discourses?
- What implicit assumptions might be shaping my questions?

We encourage our research supervisees to ask a colleague or fellow student to interview them around these questions, thus helping them to begin to question and challenge their assumptions and intentions.

## Socio-political questions

No research question can be socio-politically neutral. It is inevitably located within commonplace assumptions and premises that may be unacknowledged. For example, when we ask the following:

- What is the best treatment for people with diagnoses of personality disorders?
- Are narrative counselling therapies effective?
- Do brief therapy approaches only produce superficial changes leading to later relapse?

The first question rests on assumptions that personality disorder exists and that this is a valid way of describing a range of human experiences. Second, we need to be mindful of the possibility that interest in this is linked to political agendas, for example, policies on crime that tap into popular prejudices and fears of the 'mentally ill'. Even potentially less contentious questions regarding the value of narrative therapies can be seen to reveal important issues concerning the differences that we might ask about when we are operating from 'within' as opposed to 'outside' a therapeutic paradigm. Narrative therapists have offered some important critiques of notions of 'mental health' and the pathologizing processes inherent in any given culture. Within this paradigm it makes less sense to ask about effectiveness than to consider how clients are being freed of the pathologizing processes and labels that are entrapping them. Or, more simply, that it is not just persons but society that needs to change. The last question (concerning brief therapies) although important, makes assumptions about the process and nature of change. Also, it is highly likely that the question may be motivated by other therapies, such as psychodynamic therapies which have contended that change is a slow and painstaking process. It also possibly disguises the fact that relapse is a problem for most psychotherapies, so that brief therapies need not be singled out for such investigation.

Our point here is not that the questions above should not be explored but that this initial stage of developing questions is extremely important. If we hurry the process too much we may find later that in fact we have been asking less than helpful, or less then useful, questions. Also, it opens up the possibility that it may be helpful to give ourselves the opportunity to sharpen our questions after a preliminary investigation or 'pilot' study.

## COLLABORATIVE RESEARCH

Much of the traditional research in the social sciences, and in psychotherapy, has adopted an expert and non-collaborative approach. Typically, the researcher has generated the questions and there has been a distinct separation between the researcher and the participant. There are important ethical issues here about locating people as objects that we do research 'to' or 'on', not to mention depersonalizing people by calling them 'subjects' – a monarchistic term implying a distinct asymmetry of power. Also, we may be colluding in maintaining the 'us' and 'them' divide between 'patients' and 'therapists'. Apart from this we may be sacrificing important contributions to creativity. Surely the people that experience therapy themselves have important questions about it that are worth considering? Certainly this is supported by our own experiences of being in therapy; there are lots of interesting questions that have come to mind as a consequence of our experiences. For example, RD wanted to know what his therapist was thinking, what ideas and explanations were forming in his mind and what further questions he had. Interestingly, this kind of sharing of ideas has become central in systemic therapies which use reflecting team processes with families (Andersen, 1987).

In short, a collaborative approach is not only more respectful but also potentially adds to creativity and the validity of the study. The extent to which research may be collaborative may vary. For example, we might want to consider it being fully collaborative, with 'clients' being invited to frame the research questions and methods with us. At the other end we may want to discuss our questions with and share some of the ideas we have about the possible analysis.

## RESEARCH AIMS

All research has certain aims and intentions. Sometimes these are broad, such as an aim to advance knowledge and theory, but with the intention that this will in turn advance the effectiveness of psychotherapy to produce positive change for our clients. However, we do not usually conduct research merely for our own purposes but also to communicate our findings to others. This raises the question of the generalizability of a piece of research. Specifically, we need to consider who will read our research publications or communications and what they will be able to do with them. In effect, we need to consider from the outset not just the details of our research – design, methods, sampling, analysis and so on – but also our readership and how readers are likely to use the research findings. Such reflection may lead to recursive processes, whereby we decide to adjust our research aims and design so that the findings are more relevant and applicable to a wider group of colleagues.

Let us take a self-reflective turn for a moment. What do you do when you read a psychotherapy research report? From the outset, you might approach the paper in different ways according to whether it is a *quantitative* or *qualitative* study. However, there may be some common activities:

1  Perhaps the most immediate reaction is a broad one about applicability. This can be specific or more general. For example, what can I use from this report, say, in my next session with Jimmy and his parents when they are likely to tell me that things have been getting worse and that Jimmy and his father have had another argument, that he has smashed up the house again and has threatened his mother? Alternatively, what more general features can I extract from the report about the kinds of therapy that may suit these kinds of clients? Even more broadly, you may be less immediately interested with particular cases and more concerned with developing services.

2  The activity you are most likely to engage in will probably be linked to your role and position in the therapeutic system. If your work is predominantly as a busy therapist, your questions might be of the first sort. If you are also engaged in teaching and service development, you might be giving more weight to the less specific questions. If your role is a more managerial one, you may be less interested in specific cases and more interested in questions about types of therapy, such as whether the type of therapy described can be used to build your service within the financial constraints operating.

3  In using the report to answer any of these questions it is important to imagine the clinical population upon which the research was based. However, this is not always an easy task. Qualitative research is more likely to give such information, but not always. Despite promising to do so, it is surprising how often such information is not available.

Quantitative studies, in contrast, are less likely to offer specific idio-syncratic details but may offer information about the general character-istics of the sample in terms of statistical transformations according to measures on various clinical inventories. You may then try to estimate how much this description matches the clients that you work with.

4 Search for details of how the therapy was conducted. Again, reports may differ in how much they specify this, varying from verbatim transcripts of parts of a session or sessions, general descriptions or merely reference to the different types of therapy compared.

5 It is also likely that you will read the report within your wider system of beliefs and values about psychotherapy. For example, I will try to accommodate the findings within what I already regard as important features of therapy: a view of the importance of the therapeutic relation-ship, of taking systemic factors into account, of locating the therapy within wider socio-political contexts and so on. In contrast, it is possible that the report will offer some challenges to your assumptions, in which case you may need to re-appraise, or alter, your belief system to incorpor-ate these findings.

6 Connected to the last point, it is probably the case that many of us like to read reports that confirm, validate and support what we already do. This is not simply to bolster our prejudices. Within the painful and often despairing process of psychotherapy we may also need to seek reassurance that what we are doing is experienced and perceived to be helpful.

The chances are that in order to use the report in any of these ways we are likely to need to gather more information. We may try to assemble a range of research papers on the topic and gather further specific details from the authors, such as exactly how the therapeutic work was done. In fact often, research reports, especially quantitative reports, do not describe the therapy done in adequate detail for us to be able to judge whether they have done it in ways that are similar to our practice, unless they follow a manualized and published procedure. Interestingly, in gathering more reports together we are building a body of knowledge, or a meta-analysis, as opposed simply to using one study. There may also be times where we find some descriptions of an aspect of the therapy that is inspiring and leads us to try it. As an example, let us look at a CBT study of the fear of flying (see Research Example 2.1).

The aims of our research therefore need to fit with the activities and concerns in our reader. More broadly, we need to ask ourselves not just why we want to do the research but also what we want people to do with our findings. It could be argued that this is rather like putting the 'cart before the horse'; that an initial question that shapes our aims concerns where we intend to publish our findings and, linked to this, what conferences or work-shops we intend to offer in order to disseminate our findings. Returning to our original categories, our aims broadly fall into the following:

1 *What works*: evaluation – offering evidence about effectiveness of psycho-therapy. Often our interest here is comparative, in terms of what is the best or most effective treatment.

**Research Example 2.1**

Borrill, J. and Foreman, E. I. (1996) Understanding cognitive change: a qualitative study of the impact of cognitive-behavioural therapy on fear of flying, *Clinical Psychology and Psychotherapy*, 3(1): 62–74.

This study consisted of a series of semi-structured interviews with a group of people who had been successfully treated with a CBT approach for their fear of flying. The transcripts were analysed using a grounded theory form of analysis to elicit common themes about the experience of the therapy. A central theme was the importance of the therapeutic relationship and a sense of recognizing very early that the therapist was a helpful, kind person. One participant elegantly described this relationship as being able to 'borrow belief from the therapist'.

This phrase in particular was inspirational in how RD wanted to approach his next client. It helped to change focus from emphasizing the technique of cognitive interventions to a focus on broader issues of generating a positive approach. More broadly, the findings reported, though about CBT as the focus, helped confirm ideas about the importance of a positive solutions focused approach.

2 *How it works*: evidence about the processes of psychotherapy – what are the mechanisms and the active and vital ingredients? This can be specific exploration of any given therapeutic approach or it can be questions about common aspects, such as the therapeutic alliance.
3 *Why it works*: theoretical and conceptual issues – for example, wanting to know about the causes and developmental trajectories of various problems so that we can understand why and how the therapy works.

Inextricably bound up with our aims are questions of generalizability. We can return to our imaginary reader above and this time ask ourselves, in addition to how he or she might want to use our results, what we want to tell our reader about the details of our study, especially our sample. We need to do so in order that they have enough information to make a decision about whether our findings can be generalized to their contexts and experience. All types of psychotherapy research need to bear this in mind and we suggest one common requirement is that we specify details of our clients and their contexts in order to help readers in this process of transferring the findings to their own clients and contexts.

## GENERALIZABILITY AND TRANSFERABILITY

Arguably, generalizability is at the heart of all research. We want to be able to communicate ideas, information, evidence, findings and so on to our colleagues which they can employ to assist their own practice. We might in some cases be implying transferability. Transferability makes less forceful claims that the findings will be true to all or most situations, instead suggesting that the reader may be able to find some useful ideas and information from the findings. In psychotherapy research, generalizability is intimately connected to the core research questions we may want to ask. We will discuss these important issues later, but first we will look at some of the ways that generalizability has been considered in the areas of outcome and process research into psychotherapy.

## Evaluation and outcome study generalizations

As an example, it is frequently claimed that CBT has the strongest evidence base for the effective treatment of a variety of conditions, notably depression. This generalization is based largely on studies that have employed a randomized control trial (RCT) design. A group of people who fulfil the diagnostic criteria for depression are randomly allocated either to CBT therapy or to a group receiving, for example, standard medication and support but with no additional psychotherapy. The two groups are compared on a number of measures before and following a period of treatment and the results are subjected to statistical analysis. The construction of such a design is that if the difference between the two groups could only occur by chance less than 5 per cent of the time, then this is seen as cause to reject the null hypothesis and conclude that the differences are significant.

However, there are a number of problems and dangers in the kind of generalizations that we can draw from such studies:

- Individual differences and extreme cases. Not infrequently there will be individuals in the CBT group who do not improve or who may even get worse. Hence we cannot generalize about all people with depression.
- Often the samples are described statistically, such as average age, severity of the problem or duration of the problem. It is then difficult to generalize to the specific population we work with, or to the next client who walks through our door.
- Not infrequently the samples in such studies are unusual. For example, they may have been sifted to eliminate co-morbidity which actually may be very frequent in many clinical contexts.
- We may not know enough about the context of the study and whether the findings are applicable to the sort of situations we work in.
- The findings do not tell us very much about how and why CBT works, and hence it does not guide us in terms of ways to develop its effectiveness.

## Psychotherapy process study generalizations

One of the key intentions underlying studies of the process of psychotherapy is that we may uncover some general findings about key aspects of the process. Perhaps the most significant of such general findings has been that the therapeutic relationship is a key ingredient in most therapies, even if it is not specifically identified as such in the theory that informs the therapy.

Some studies have employed group data, for example, by rating assessments by a group of clients about their relationships with their therapist and comparing this to outcome. Another approach has been to interview groups of people about their experience and draw out general themes which capture the details of the experience. In contrast to group studies, single case studies have also been used to reveal how the therapeutic relationship evolves and changes, the expectations of the clients and therapist, differences in their perceptions and so on. In addition, this allows nuances and details of their relationship to be described.

Single case studies may be a counter to some of the difficulties relating to group designs described above. However, they also contain their own problems:

- It may be tempting to overgeneralize to cases which do not match those described.
- We have no way of knowing whether the effects found do apply to different therapist–client pairings.
- We do not know whether what is described as helpful and so on by one client might not be described as quite unhelpful by another.

## Nomothetic versus idiographic approach

Broadly, there is a distinction between an *idiographic* and *nomothetic* approach. An idiographic approach seeks to capture the complexity and uniqueness of, for example, a clinical approach, such as how clients and therapists might experience the process of CBT. In contrast, a nomothetic approach is more concerned in making generalizations, such as that CBT is *generally* effective for people suffering with depression. The latter might be the sort of information that managers and purchasers of services want, whereas the former might be what interests clinicians, in terms of how the therapy is experienced, how it works and so on.

Debates have raged, with qualitative and idiographic approaches usually placed in the same camp and with arguments that we can only experience the world through our personal, subjective lenses. Further criticism has in turn revolved around arguments that this kind of research raises questions (and answers) that are not objective and remain essentially personal with non-generalizable results. Alternatively, nomothetic approaches have been seen to argue that there is a real world which we can measure, quantify and predict and that this prompts research that produces objective and generalizable data and theory. Rather than becoming stuck on this unhelpful polarization, we want to suggest that a reflective approach allows us to work within both orientations.

More fundamentally, generalizability connects with more profound questions of knowledge and epistemology. These terms are employed to distinguish between research which aims to produce general laws that are universally true (nomothetic) and research which attempts to understand particular events (idiographic). It has been argued that the polarizations propounded in the current usage of these terms contains a misinterpretation of the original meaning of the terms, which were coined by Windleband (1921). By nomothetic, apparently he meant knowledge which is always true or covered by the generalization being made. However, in the study of human beings and in counselling and psychotherapy we can only verify such a generalization by looking at individual cases. So, if we claim that CBT is effective for the treatment of depression, we need to explore individuals receiving treatment and find explanations for why it does not work in some cases. So nomethetic knowledge does not simply come out of group comparisons based on statistical inference. The study of individuals can add to an understanding of how common, general factors play out in individual cases. Such knowledge adds to, or thickens, and enriches the nomothetic research. Allport (1962) further emphasized that idiographic research, as well as nomothetic, requires a concern with reliability and prediction. Investigation of individual cases is not based on intuition but is subject to the same rigorous gathering and testing of data, for example, observations of a therapeutic case involving data from the therapist, client and investigator(s).

More broadly, it has been variously argued that attempts at basing psychology on a limited model of research developed in the natural sciences has in many ways been a misguided enterprise. One of the core reasons for this is that our knowledge may develop very little without an understanding of the reasons behind people's behaviour:

> Billy cuts a worm in half because Billy has a sadistic streak. Jimmy cuts a worm in half so that, with two, the worm will no longer be lonely. A 'paradigm' that features the outcome and ignores the rationale must miss everything that is of real importance, even as it painstakingly strives for accuracy in measurement and merely statistical 'significance'.
>
> (Robinson, 2000, p. 42)

This is not to claim that psychological research should not employ numbers or attempt to make nomothetic generalizations, but this should not be at the expense of the individual. In fact, when we say 'individual' we can also add here relational systems, such as couples, families and groups that also may have some commonalities as well as individual characteristics. It can be argued that the detailed study of single cases or small groups of individuals can offer more in the way of testing, exploring and refining theory than studies based on statistical inference:

> I believe that the almost universal reliance on merely refuting the null hypothesis as the standard method for corroborating substantive theories is . . . one of the worst things that ever happened in the history of psychology.
>
> (Meehl, 1978, p. 817)

Part of the problem is that the kind of theory that it is possible to develop on the basis of comparisons of groups, even when statistically significant, does not promote development of theory or understanding to any significant degree. Especially in the context of psychotherapy, even though group comparisons may give some general indications that an approach works, our knowledge of how and why it works may not be extended significantly.

Lamiel (1998) argues further that part of the underlying problem is that psychology has confused the idea of 'aggregate' with 'general'. If, for example, we talk about how overall, on average, a group of people performed as a result of a piece of psychodynamic therapy, we need not become consumed with making statements about what might be true for every person. Furthermore, we can then develop a proper science of psychology and psychotherapy that allows us to talk about aggregates and fully accept that there are individual differences making up this aggregate. Studying these different cases gives us a fuller scientific picture, which allows us to talk about aggregate findings along with an analysis of each person's history, circumstances and so on.

## The search for meaning

The search for meaning links with a further set of epistemological issues relating to generalizability. Perhaps it is fair to argue that psychotherapy research needs to take account of meaning in human life. After all, people come to therapy with significant issues that are problematic in their life. But underlying these is the sense that their lives are not as they should be; that life does not make sense, seems unfair and is unfulfilled; in short, that life is often lacking in meaning and direction. Though there are still ongoing debates here, few therapists would argue that a therapy which does not address meanings is sufficient. Behavioural approaches have in the past largely bypassed a consideration of meanings, but even here it surely must be conceded that the very fact that someone comes for any form of therapy suggests a set of underlying meanings in place, something along the lines of: 'I want, can, could, should feel better than I do.' In some cases people are still 'sent' for therapy by family and friends, but it is likely that they too will have ideas about this: 'It's not really my problem, it's theirs.' An ability to express this may in fact be a vital ingredient for the therapy to be helpful.

The broader issue here is between constructivist and positivist views of the world. In relation to research in psychotherapy, the question can be put simply in terms of ontology and epistemology.

Ontology is concerned with what we believe is real, what is seen to be the essence of clinical problems. For example, we can hold the view that problems are to do with neurologically based deficits. In this sense they exist as real biochemical events and activities. Alternatively, we may believe that problems exist as clusters of meanings that are attributed to aspects of our lives.

Epistemology, on the other hand, is concerned with how we discover how and why problems occur. An important contrast here is between a positivist and constructivist epistemology. A positivist epistemology is where we believe that an objective approach is possible and where we attempt to develop our knowledge by using standardized measures and instruments. Alternatively, a constructivist epistemology is that knowledge progresses through understandings. Problems are not predominantly or simply objective entities but constellations of meanings that we can move towards understanding by interacting with and engaging with clients.

Though stated simply above, this broadly encapsulates important issues regarding the questions that we start to generate about psychotherapy and our views of the generalizability of our findings. Further to this, Hamlyn (1970) describes four epistemological positions that relate to these two positions:

1 *Correspondence theory of truth* – a belief is true if it matches reality. This is a position from a realist or positivist view in that it supports the idea that there is a reality 'out there' which we need to and can investigate, measure and map. A theory is seen as needing to match reality.

2 *Pragmatic or utilitarian theory* – a theory is useful or produces practical benefits. This view places less emphasis on the real world and more on the reality of consequences. In a sense it is less concerned with absolute truth of a theory than with the effects of a theory.

3 *Coherence theory* – a belief is true if it is internally consistent or logically non-contradictory. This is based on a view that suggests that there is not a real world out there but there is such a thing as rational thinking and argument. The processes of our minds, especially logic, are what can be considered real.

4 *Consensual* – a belief is true if it is shared by a group of people. This adopts an inter-subjective view of knowledge and suggests that a theory or belief is true if it is upheld by a group of people. In effect the only things that are real are the shared understandings between people.

(Adapted from Barker *et al.*, 1994, p. 11)

Theories 1 and 2 are based in a more positivist framework, which views the world as an objective entity and sees the task of research as being to accurately and objectively describe this. It has also been referred to as a 'critical realist' view, which embraces much of psychological research (Cook and Campbell, 1979). This assumes that there is a real world out there, though we can never know it with total certainty. Our understandings are tentative, but nevertheless it is assumed that we are approaching this reality and that our findings are generalizable.

Theories 3 and 4 make less claims about reality. Rather, the view is that the world, certainly of therapy, is to do with meanings and understandings. We can attempt to explore these but the attempt is not to arrive at some ultimate truth.

Each of the four epistemological positions can be seen to be inadequate by itself. Correspondence theory involves an infinite regression, in that reality must be measured validly before we can assess the degree of correspondence. With coherence theory we can imagine an elegant theory which has no basis in reality; we can imagine a pragmatic theory which is false but useful, and a consensual theory which is based on a form of shared or social delusion. Arguably, all four of these criteria are necessary to construct a convincing research epistemological position (Elliott *et al.*, 1994).

These epistemological positions have serious implications for how we think about our study contributing to knowledge and clinical practice. We will turn to specific examples of sampling in Chapter 3, as well as further discussion of the issue of generalizability in qualitative research, where this issue has to some extent become blurred or even dismissed.

## DO-ABLE RESEARCH

Part of the exploration of the research questions needs to involve some hard thinking about the practicalities of the research. A particular issue for clinical research is who our participants will be, where they are and how we will be able to invite them into the research (see also Chapter 3). In taking a collaborative stance, we may have started to address these questions since our participants are with us from the start. Nevertheless, it is frequently the case in psychotherapy research that we are interested in exploring relatively uncommon and relatively unique experiences, such as research into the effectiveness of psychotherapy with young sex offenders or attachment oriented family therapy with young people with anorexia. In both of these possible pieces of research, researchers have found considerable difficulty in recruiting participants. Often we are in a position of needing to adopt an 'opportunistic sampling approach' (see Chapter 3), whereby the research sample is determined largely by who is available to take part. This alters the kinds of questions we are able to ask and the kinds of generalizations that we might intend to result from our research:

- *Exploratory research questions.* For many clinicians attempting a piece of research, it is possible that the kinds of questions that they are able to address are exploratory, in that they may offer some initial ideas about the questions initially inspired by the two examples above.
- *Local questions.* The types of questions that we may be able to ask are relatively local. We may be able to generate some ideas about the populations that we work with, but these may not be so easily generalizable across all contexts, for example with therapy for young offenders or clinicians attempting to employ attachment ideas with family therapy for eating disorders. Such groups of clients may also vary according to regional differences and the nature of services and their criteria for offering treatments.

What we are suggesting is that there is an important recursive process between thinking about our research aims and thinking about the practicalities of the research. Of course, clinicians may be able to be a part of larger studies, for example larger controlled studies. There are important issues here too. Though it may be possible to recruit a bigger sample, it is a risk that we then lose the ability to gain insights into the experience and nature of the psychotherapy. Consequently, it may become harder to translate the findings to our own local clinical practice.

Finally, we are also able to gain some ideas about the do-ableness of our research aims by looking at the available literature as part of our literature review. If we look closely, some studies reveal the resources, cost and time that went into the study. We can also glean some information about the difficulties of recruitment, such as how many people were approached to take part and how many dropped out of the study. Sometimes, such drop-out is hard to predict. In one recent study comparing family therapy, medication and CBT for depression (Jones and Asen, 2000), such a large proportion of clients dropped out of the CBT part of the trials that these could no longer be included in the study. This was a serious problem for a major piece of research involving considerable funding, time and effort.

## THE LITERATURE REVIEW

The literature review has two main purposes: to support both the development of the research question and the analysis of the findings (Hart, 2000). In the field of psychotherapy research there are many competing models and research designs. The complexity of our psychotherapy world places a strong requirement on us to be clear and rigorous in our approach to the literature review. There are different approaches to conducting a literature review. For example, you might review all the empirical data in the area of your enquiry, both supportive and contradictory; you might review all the conceptual literature to identify directions for research; you might review existing research designs for their utility in approaching the question(s) of interest; and/or you might review all policy related research literature to identify key implications for practice. Clearly, the literature review needs to be linked to the overall aims of the research. This might involve taking a within discipline or multidisciplinary perspective, a national or international perspective, a within culture or cross-culture perspective, and so on.

We recommend that students write the rationale for their literature review before starting, to show how they are thinking about the overall place and purpose of the literature review in their research enterprise. The rationale should consider the following:

1  What is the contribution of the literature review to the aims of the research, and how will it support the development of the research question? (Or is it designed to identify and hone the research question?)
2  What is the main focus of the review and why? (Will this include identifying key papers – experimental and/or theoretical – to which other related, less crucial papers can be connected?)
3  Where will the review be positioned in the various stages of the research? (For example, will the review be done in two parts, where the first part supports the development of the research question, and the second part, done during the research analysis, helps make sense of the findings and locates them in the context of other literatures, much as in a grounded theory study?)
4  How will the conclusions from the literature review be integrated with the conclusions from the research? (For example, will the conclusions from the literature review be used as part of a triangulation strategy to explore the validity of the study?)

Once the rationale for the literature review has been agreed, it is then necessary to think about how it will be achieved. Clearly, the rationale above presupposes some of the 'how', but a detailed plan for how it will be conducted that includes search sites, means of searching, identification of key words and concepts, resources needed and the time scale is important. It helps us think about what we shall include in the review, and what we shall exclude, and why. Once the outer boundaries have been agreed, we can think of the shape of the review: an inner circle of key papers, with outer concentric rings of decreasing importance; or connected concepts, like a thought map or eco map; or a Venn diagram of overlapping circles. The initial search needs to be as comprehensive as possible, according to our identified concepts, and then focused according to our plan.

Hart (2000) has written extensively about literature reviewing in social science research. We hope that the following points, based on our experience as research supervisors, will prove helpful:

- Do not forget to critique the literature you review, both research and theoretical work, in terms of its relative strengths and weaknesses. We find that people we have supervised sometimes do not say what they like about research or theory, and why they like it, almost as if they are too shy to venture an opinion. For example, when critiquing both research and theory, are the concepts clear and operationally defined? Is it clear how the concepts are related to each other? Can the concepts be observed, measured, and/or tested?
- Include the author's own voice: their hunches, suggestions and speculations. Comment on these from your own perspective and what your clinical experience has taught you.
- Make connections where you can between the different sections of the literature you have reviewed, showing how these connections support the development of your research question.
- Make sure you are clear as to why you have reviewed some studies and not others, given that you have to be selective and cannot always review everything. Have you identified a handful of key studies and/or theoretical reviews that are central to the development of your research question?
- What are the gaps in your literature review? Do you need to tell your reader why they are there?
- Make sure that your literature review 'walks' your reader towards your research question(s), almost as if the research literature reviewed funnels down to the research question. In this way, the reader understands how the research question seems to arise 'naturally' from the foregoing discussion. Careful reading of your argument at this stage is important.
- Finally, when approaching the writing of your discussion section, do not forget to locate the discussion of your findings in the extant literature, reviewed in your introduction. You should examine how your findings complement those of other researchers and how the analysis of your findings led you on to discover other research literature.

## KEY REFERENCES

Allport, G. W. (1962) *The Person in Psychology: Selected Essays*. Boston: Beacon Press.

Barker, C., Pistrang, N. and Elliott, R. (2002) *Research Methods in Clinical and Counselling Psychology*. Chichester: Wiley.

Cook, T. D. and Campbell, D. T. (1979) *Quasi-experimentation: Design and Analysis for Field Settings*. Chicago: Rand-McNally.

Elliott, R., Fischer, C. T. and Rennie, D. L. (1999) Evolving guidelines for publication of qualitative research studies in psychology and related fields, *British Journal of Clinical Psychology*, 38: 215–29.

Hamlyn, D. W. (1970) *The Theory of Knowledge*. Garden City, NY: Doubleday-Anchor.

Hart, C. (2000) *Doing a Literature Review: Releasing the Social Science Research Imagination*. London: Sage.

Meehl, P. (1978) Theoretical risks and tabular asterisks: Sir Karl, Sir Ronald, and the slow progress of soft psychology, *Journal of Consulting and Clinical Psychology*, 26: 806–34.

Popper, K. R. (1959) *The Logic of Scientific Discovery*. New York: Basic Books. (Original German edition 1934.)

# 3    SAMPLING AND GENERALIZABILITY

## CHAPTER OVERVIEW

This chapter is based on the view that research often starts with the important question of who our research will focus on: who will the research be about? In clinical research this is often framed initially in terms of an interest in particular types of problems, clients and treatments.

The chapter starts with a discussion of the key role of sampling in the research process. It argues that decisions about sampling are intimately connected with the research questions. Comparisons and contrasts are drawn between research where the sample is chosen to test an existing theory and that where people are chosen in order to develop our understanding. Specific issues regarding sampling in clinical research are considered, especially the use of small, extreme and heterogenous samples. Sampling in quantitative and qualitative research is compared and connections are drawn to questions of generalizability, discussed in more detail in

Chapters 2 and 10. Qualitative research is discussed further and sampling considerations for case study and small group research are outlined (see also Chapter 7).

## QUESTIONS OF SAMPLING

Sampling is arguably one of the key issues in any piece of research. It is fundamental to the framing of our research questions and, importantly, to the question of the applications of our research findings. Specifically, it is centrally connected to the issue of generalizability. The characteristics of our sample determine what use can be made of our findings.

In quantitative research the general assumption has been that a sample is chosen such that *nomothetic* (universal) generalizations can be made. An example might be research of CBT (cognitive behaviour therapy) for depression, where it has been assumed that by using a sample of clients who correspond to the definitions of clinical depression as measured by the BDI II (Beck Depression Inventory) the findings will be generalizable to all clients who meet this criteria in various clinical settings. Not infrequently in fact, such studies become overgeneralized to the point that it is assumed that CBT will also be the most effective treatment for a whole range of other emotional conditions. By way of contrast, in qualitative studies the approach has been *idiographic*, in that the interest is more in a deep, or thick, description, such as what the experience of CBT is like.

Nevertheless, readers of both types of research will attempt to do something with the findings. The rich idiographic description, for example, might lead a clinician to reflect on his or her own practice and resolve to try to be more sensitive to a client's needs for reassurance and encouragement early in therapy when change is possible. Reading a nomothetic study we might resolve to convince our manager that it is worth investing in staffing or training in CBT to develop a service for a client group with depression.

### Deductive and inductive sampling

Corresponding to the differences between nomothetic and idiographic research is the idea that our sampling is deductively guided by a body of theory rather than an aim to inductively develop some theory. In psychotherapy and counselling research, the theory may be that a particular approach – again, for example, that CBT will be effective not just for depression but also for anxiety – was based on a theoretical understanding of emotional problems which stressed that these were shaped by 'negative automatic thought processes'. Hence, by a process of deduction, treatment for anxiety based on some of the same principles as those for depression *should* work. In this we are making a prediction and then seeking to identify a group of people – our sample – which can adequately test this prediction. In order to do so the sample will need to contain a set of characteristics that we can define, for example, a level of anxiety. We may then choose to make a broad generalization by having a broad sample which contains people of various ages, gender, ethnicity, length of suffering with the problem, absence of other problems and so on, so that our findings will be widely generalizable.

By contrast, in an idiographic approach our sampling is based on an inductive approach, in that we may be hoping that some understanding or theory may emerge from our research. However, it is not initially guided by theory. The first stage is to gain description and understanding, usually of what the experience means for participants. So, in the example above, this will involve finding out what clients undergoing CBT for anxiety may feel about the experience. What do they make of the therapy? What do they find helpful? What sense do they make of the tasks, such as diary keeping? We will discuss this in more detail later, but we can note that our sampling might, therefore, be based on selecting a small number of people who are going through an experience, such as CBT for anxiety, and gaining an in-depth picture of the experience for them.

This partly depends on whether such exploratory studies have been pre-viously attempted. If they have, we might refine our sampling somewhat to contain certain characteristics, such as gender, or to focus on certain age bands, severity levels or on people for whom the treatment has worked very well as opposed to those for whom it has not. However, this is in the knowledge that our sampling will not be testing an embracing theory although it might elaborate or illuminate theory. It is nevertheless impor-tant to consider these questions carefully in qualitative research. Not infrequently what may happen is that the sample is shaped by service or diagnostic factors. Thus by default we have a selective sample based not on what we intended to study but, for example, on the fact that this is the only type of treatment available and that some clients feel that they had very little choice. This would then provide a distorted picture of what the experience is like for them.

So questions regarding sampling, the research questions and aims are intimately connected. For example, often the research questions start with an interest in looking at people who have a particular condition or who are experiencing a particular form of treatment, or often a combination of the two. As we proceed, the questions regarding the research aims and the sampling may simultaneously become more specific, such as an interest in looking at people who are experiencing a problem or are in distress but as yet have not been formally diagnosed, have not yet received treatment or are on a waiting list. This serves to spell out further the characteristics of the research sample and it applies to both qualitative and quantitative research.

In qualitative research there may subsequently be a greater emphasis on exploring individual as well as shared characteristics of the participants, but some initial decision has to be made about what the sample will be. In case study research this may be a very small sample of one, but then there is an even greater need to think about why this person is chosen. Connecting to our earlier discussion in Chapters 1 and 2, we have to be careful that implicit assumptions do not slip in at this stage. For example, as a matter of expediency we might go for a sample based on diagnostic criteria which may assume an organic or medical view of the problems we want to study. However, we may choose this approach in part because much of the prior research has done so. Roth and Fonagy (1996) argue that the reason why much research on psychotherapy continues to employ the DSM and ICD diagnostic systems is that it allows a connection with the extant literature.

In Fig. 3.1 (from Barker *et al.*, 1994) it is possible to think of sampling in terms of identifying a target population that constitutes the people we are interested in studying. This may be to do with types of problems, types of clients, types of therapies and so on. This group can be seen as residing within a wider population and, in turn, the wider universe. The critical issue is how we draw out a sample of people for our study which can tell us something useful about the target population in which we are interested.

- *Probability sampling*: this is also often defined as random sampling, and involves drawing participants from the target population in a random way, for example one in ten of every suitable client.
- *Stratified sampling:* this involves selecting people on the basis of some specified variables, for example, on the basis of gender, social class and severity of problems.
- *Convenience sampling:* this is where essentially we study whomever is available. Often in clinical contexts it may be that this is a pragmatic limitation that we have to accept. However, there are a number of related issues that may lead us to accept an essentially convenience sample:
  1 Participants are not easily available
  2 Participants do not fall into neat groupings according to variables
  3 Participants may be at extreme ends of our variables.

### Extreme cases

Clinicians are typically working with extreme parts of populations. For example, in many group or randomized design studies the statistical 'outliers' at the extremes of the distribution may be rejected from the sample because they distort it. However, these 'extreme' cases may be just the people that psychotherapists are most interested in. They may be the clients who are difficult to produce any change with, have a multiplicity of

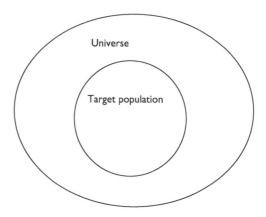

**Figure 3.1**   Sampling as a population drawn from the wider universe

problems and are hard to engage in therapy (Vetere and Myers, 2004). Arguably, research which excludes this group is ultimately not very helpful in guiding our work with this more difficult group who typically consume a lot of our time and resources.

A powerful example of this issue has been the study by Jones and Asen (2000) which compared CBT, systemic couples therapy and drug therapy for people with depression. It was found that over 80 per cent of the clients in the CBT arm of the trial dropped out prematurely and that this was almost certainly due to the nature of recruitment into the study – of willingness to be randomly assigned to any of the three treatments of the study – which served to recruit the more seriously depressed people:

> 'to accept the conditions of the study probably means that one has given up hope for oneself'. However, despite its widely acclaimed success with depression CBT has in fact only established its success with depression of recent onset and of short duration.
>
> (Jones and Asen, 2000)

## Bias processes

There are various processes that may affect the sample that we end up with. For example, participants who volunteer to take part may be different to those who do not. In psychotherapy research it may be the case that clients who have a reasonably good relationship with their therapist may agree to take part. In some cases people who are disaffected with a service may not wish to take part unless they see it as an opportunity to criticize services. There may also be situations where a participant takes part – for example, in a qualitative study – in order to justify or defend their position, such as research with people who have committed acts of abuse. This highlights the need from the very outset of a piece of research to think about our participants in terms of their understandings, beliefs and expectations. In fact it may be the case that some of the kinds of clients we most need to research are least likely to take part.

### *Availability and motivation*

Related to the above issue is the question of getting hold of our participants. Many clinicians describe just how difficult this can be. One reason may be the relatively small number of clients who fit particular criteria, for example, enough people entering a service who are hearing voices. In practice it is not uncommon for there to be fewer people available who fit our criteria than had initially been hoped. Also, some participants may helpfully agree to participate but may be overtaken by complex life events so that they become unavailable or cannot reliably attend.

In addition to being interested in exploring how particular therapies work and their effectiveness, we are interested in issues relating to specific populations. To take an example, one of us (RD) has worked with families where a young member is suffering with anorexia nervosa. He was interested in exploring what aspects of their emotional dynamics were relevant to family therapy and how the therapy might need to be adapted in order to meet their needs. Partly this interest was fuelled by the clinical observation that engaging in reflexive conversations about relationships, feelings and others' internal states often appeared to be difficult for these families. A piece of qualitative research was initiated to explore these issues. He had predicted from his clinical work that families might have some anxiety about taking part but had underestimated this and experienced immense difficulty in persuading them to take part. One approach that proved to be effective was to build on the trust that clinical colleagues had been able to develop in their work with the families. Reassurance, clarification and some encouragement from their therapist helped to enlist families into the research, which they subsequently found to be a positive experience and less threatening than therapy.

Sampling issues and choice of design may also be interconnected. There may be cases where we wish to explore with clients who will not engage in therapy or research, for example, young men who behave aggressively. Though unlikely to be able to engage these young men in interview types of research we may be able to conduct an observational study with them. It is important to note that research on why people do not engage in psychotherapy is important, possibly as important as research with people who are willing to do so. Arguably, some of the most complex cases, and people who represent a high risk and cost to society, are just such a group who, not surprisingly, we know the least about!

## Homogenous and heterogenous samples

One of the first questions we need to ask, and typically one of the primary questions in any research, is about our target population. Who is the study intended to be concerned with? For example, we might be initially interested in wanting to study the effectiveness of CBT with depressed young people who offend. This specifies our research population but we also need to address some general dimensions, such as gender, class, type of offending, age, severity of depression, living situation and ethnicity.

A *homogenous sample* is when we define our population of interest very specifically. The central idea is that we reduce the degree of extraneous variables, which presumably allows us to focus on the effects that we are interested in. In quantitative research this is called reducing the variance due to other factors.

On the other hand, a *heterogenous sample* is when our population is much less narrowly defined. For example, we might be interested in gender differences in depression. This could include people that differ on all of the broad variables, such as class and ethnicity, listed above.

Barker *et al.* (1994) outline some of the cost and benefits in adopting a narrowly homogenous sample:

1 *Reduced generalizability* – our ability to extend our findings may be reduced; for example, if we study adolescent offenders we may not be able to generalize to adults. It may also be the case that if we have a very narrow population it almost becomes clinically meaningless; for

example, many research studies employ participants with distinct diagnostic criteria. Yet, in common clinical practice our clients are likely to be co-morbid, vary in their circumstances and so on.

2 *Pragmatic difficulties* – these are critical for clinical research. The more strict and narrow our inclusion criteria the harder we might find it to recruit participants. Since clinical populations are often distressed, in difficulty and struggling with a variety of practical problems, we can expect that they may not turn up, may drop out of the research and so on. In the context of limited time available for many research projects, especially on psychotherapy and counselling training courses this can be a major problem.

3 *Individual differences* – we may be interested not only in our key criterion – for example, depression – but also in some individual differences connected with this, such as gender or age.

Alternatively, if our sample is too broad:

1 We cannot be sure that the effects are due to the variable(s) of interest
2 It will be difficult to generalize our findings
3 Development of any coherent theory will be difficult
4 It will be difficult for other clinicians to determine how the results and our sample can apply to their clinical context.

What may be helpful is to employ samples that are somewhere between the two extremes, although the extent to which they lean towards homogeneity or heterogeneity needs detailed consideration (see Fig. 3.2).

## Sample size

Though not wishing to perpetuate the qualitative/quantitative research divide, for the sake of clarity we will consider sample size issues separately for a moment.

### Quantitative studies

We will briefly review some concepts regarding sample size here. There are many good accounts (Barker *et al.*, 2002) from which some of the following summary is taken.

It has been a general assumption that the larger the sample size the better, since the variance due to extraneous variables becomes comparatively less in relation to the variance due to the effects that we are interested in.

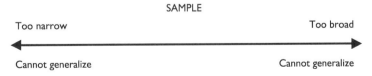

Figure 3.2

However, the picture is a little more complicated than this. Using too large a sample can be a waste of effort and, importantly, may reveal trivial effects. Importantly in psychotherapy research, we generally need effects to be quite large in order for them to have clinical significance. Fishing for statistically significant results is unhelpful.

### Statistical power

The statistical power of a study is the likelihood that it will detect an effect that is present. High power means that there is a good chance that the study will detect the effect if it is present, while low power means that it is unlikely to detect it. If the study is not powerful enough, important effects may be ignored. Consideration of statistical power is based on calculating both the probabilities of Type 1 and Type 2 errors:

- Type 1 Error $\alpha$ (false positive) – the probability of finding an effect, which could have occurred by chance. In psychological research this has conventionally been set at 5 per cent (or $p < 0.05$).
- Type 2 Error $\beta$ (false negative) – the probability of missing an effect which is present.

Statistical power is defined as $1-\beta$, which is the probability of detecting an effect that is really there. It is usually recommended that this be 0.8, which means that there should be an 80 per cent chance of detecting an effect that is there.

Calculating statistical power consists of four steps:

1 Effect size. This is the size of the effect that we are studying, for example, the change in scores on depression produced by a course of CBT. A large effect size is one that is very obvious and does not need statistical analysis. Effect sizes are usually classified into large, medium and small effects. Arguably a small effect size is often not of a great deal of interest in clinical research. Effect size is calculated according to the statistical test that is to be employed; for example, in correlational studies a Pearson correlation coefficient of 0.10 is considered small, 0.30 medium and 0.50 a large effect. The calculation is based on the sampling distributions (see Cohen, 1988).
2 Select the statistical power level ($\beta$). This is usually set at 0.80.
3 Select your level of significance ($\alpha$). This is usually $p < 0.05$.
4 Look in power calculation tables, or a computer program, e.g. G.Power, to calculate the sample size required.

As an example, in a study which compares two groups using a t-test, with medium effect sizes and an $\alpha$ of 0.05, a sample of 32 people per group is required. Barker *et al.* (2002) point out that the sample size requirements for studies that attempt to compare therapies are so large that they should only be attempted with adequate funding and staffing. This suggests that for smaller-scale projects this is not viable. Research ethics committees have also generally taken the position that studies with inadequate sample sizes will not be passed because they are unethical. This is on the grounds that they are unlikely to produce statistically significant results and, therefore, will be a waste of the participants' time.

## QUALITATIVE RESEARCH

As we have discussed, qualitative studies typically adopt an idiographic approach which emphasizes the uniqueness of phenomena rather than seeking to make nomothetic (broad universal) generalizations. In case study research, obviously the sample size in many cases will be N=1 and we will discuss in the final section some of the criteria we may choose in selecting a case. However, many qualitative studies involve group studies. As discussed earlier, typically studies take an inductive approach, in that we are not attempting to test theories but rather to develop or build understanding. A qualitative study may utilize one relatively homogenous group or in some cases attempt to compare two groups which contrast in some key factor, for example, to identify differences in accounts of childhood experiences of violent and non-violent, young offenders.

### Sample size

Advice regarding sample sizes for qualitative research has varied. Some studies have employed sample sizes equivalent to quantitative studies, while at the other extreme there are the single case studies. One guideline is that the minimum for a group qualitative study should be no less than five participants (Smith *et al.*, 1999). The decision regarding sample size is no longer based on statistical calculations but may include some of the following:

1 *Mental capacity*. This is concerned with the researcher's ability to analyse and synthesise detailed accounts from participants. If we interview say 20 people, it is not possible both to hold in mind the unique characteristics of each participant and to draw out some general themes. One argument is that the limit of our mental capacity to hold complex ideas in mind at once is about 7 (+ or −2) and for this reason our sample size needs to stay within the limits of what we can usefully make sense of (Smith *et al.*, 1999). There are examples of research which employ qualitative methods, using semi-structured interviews, but on such a large sample (100+) the results can only be presented in the form of content analysis or frequency tables with statistical comparisons. Arguably, this defeats the purpose of qualitative research which aims to capture both uniqueness of meanings relating to a phenomenon as well as commonalities.
2 *Homogeneity of the sample*. As in quantitative research our sample may be quite varied and heterogeneous due, for example, to pragmatic constraints of recruiting participants in clinical contexts. This may mean that we want to group our participants in terms of one or more variables, such as gender, age and so on. In this case it is necessary to increase the sample size so that we have roughly 5+ in each of these groups. This will also apply, of course, if our original design was a comparative one.

3 *Demands for generalizability*. In a recent study, using in-depth interviews, Stephen Frosh and colleagues (2000) explore with boys (and a sample of girls) their ideas about masculinity. Since the intention of this project was to comment on the 'crisis of masculinity', and the study was substantially funded to address this question, the sample needed to be large in order to be able legitimately to comment on this issue. A sample of over 100 boys from a range of class backgrounds, ethnicity, types of schooling and so on were recruited into the study. Not untypically in studies using such large samples, the presentation of the results is based on a relatively small number of cases with the other results offered as corroborative background information.

## Case study research

We will discuss case study research in Chapter 7. However, the sampling issues apply in case studies relating to the choice of cases. A central issue is the relationship of the case to the phenomenon that we wish to study:

- *Exemplars or prototypical cases*. One approach is to choose a case which is in some sense an exemplar or prototypical of the phenomena we want to study. This involves making some assumptions about what is typical. In clinical work, however, the range may be relatively narrow, for example the types of clients we work with. We may then also make a broader assumption that this is representative of the types of cases the consumers of our research are involved with. To facilitate this we may want to add information about, for example, the types of problems, clients and services that the particular case study may be relevant to. This approach requires us to be quite specific in our assumptions and to actively seek out cases that we think are typical.
- *Naturalistic case studies/thick description*. This approach involves less of an attempt to state what we think is typical. The case is likely to fall broadly within the domain of interest. The assumption then is that by offering details of clients, contexts, nature of the therapy and rich descriptions, our reader can decide to what extent it is similar or different to their own work and, by comparison and contrast, be able to make generalizations.
- *Intrinsic interest*. This approach to case studies resides in a view that some cases are interesting in their own right, for example, a particular service with the recognition that the findings may not necessarily be generalizable to other services. As an example, a UK NHS Trust may wish to know how the addition of a day-treatment programme in an adolescent in-patient unit has progressed without an aim that this will be of relevance or generalizable to other contexts.

An important feature of case study research is that the application of the findings is seen to be relevant to the researcher and potentially to readers of the findings. The research questions come from both a personal as well as a more generalizable interest. To take another example, we may be interested in the particular kind of problems experienced by a client. It is of interest to us as clinicians to know something specifically about this client's experience. At the same time we can see her as representing some key characteristics which are common to types of problem which might be relevant to various clinical contexts. This might be a young woman who has experienced sexual abuse as an important factor in her eating disorder. Our interest may be in how she responds to Cognitive Analytical Therapy and the details of the nature of this experience for her. If she can be seen to represent some common features of women who have had such experiences we can generalize from the account of her therapy as well as take account of how some of her unique aspects interact with the therapy.

A single case may also be selected to *test* a particular theory or generalization. For example, we may want to test whether certain family configurations underlie the development of self-harm in young women. If we find a case where these dynamics are absent but the problem is present or the opposite, this may help us to revise our explanations of how such a problem is caused.

## Theoretical sampling

This is an approach which can be employed in single case methods or in group designs. It has been rigorously articulated in the qualitative research approach of Grounded Theory. Here, sampling develops alongside emerging theory. To start with, a 'typical' instance of the phenomenon of interest is selected, for example, a person's experience of hearing voices and their account of its development. Following an analysis of this first case – typically this is of the transcript from a first interview – some preliminary ideas or hypotheses may be developed. This may suggest that distressing family experiences are central. In order to pursue this line of thinking further, a case is selected based on this emerging theory, for example, where the person appears to have had little in the way of distressing family experiences. Analysis of this case may indicate that it is the extent to which family experiences can be openly discussed, as opposed to denied, which unites the two cases. This leads to the choice of the next case where family communication appears to be more open. Choices of whom, and how many people, to include in the sample are made in an ongoing way until no new features are apparent. The sample size, therefore, cannot be determined in advance.

## Generalizability in qualitative research

To conclude this section we need to return to the issue of generalizability in qualitative research. The processes and rationale for generalization have been widely articulated in quantitative research and these are often used to castigate qualitative research. Unfortunately, there has been inadequate discussion of generalizability in qualitative research, partly in an attempt to distance it from some of the problems of positivist quantitative research. Yet this can be a substantial mistake. To form generalizations is arguably a fundamental human activity and Gomm *et al.* (2000) make the point that people tend to make generalizations from their everyday observations. They also add that these generalizations are prone to error. However, in order to make sense of our world we need to be able to categorize our experiences and the wider world, and part of this process is that we expect some of these categorizations to have some durability and to exist across situations and time. For example, when two therapists discuss their cases they will make connections and will draw out commonalities in their experience: 'Oh yes, I saw a family just like that'; or 'That does seem to happen a lot with cases of anorexia.' It does injustice to both research and to everyday conversation to frame such exchanges as merely anecdotal.

### Theoretical versus empirical generalization

It is possible to develop generalizations from research based on a detailed description of a case or a group of interviews. Such small-scale research findings can be employed to generate modest, tentative theoretical frameworks. This requires the reader to make some connections and draw out possible generalizations to their own context. Much qualitative research can stay at this level of generalizability and does not make bigger claims to develop a more formal theory. This would consist of extrapolating from the findings to make more ambitious claims of offering an encompassing theory.

As an example, Goffman (1961) generated a theory about the nature of the functioning of asylums from his case study of an asylum, with his idea of the 'total institution', whereby all aspects of patients' lives become structured and constructed by the hospital. He suggested that such organizations operate out of expediency and the needs of the staff, such that it is easier to provide ready-made food rather than to encourage inmates to cook for themselves since this is more time consuming, expensive, dangerous and so on. Consequently, the therapeutic needs to promote independence, self-respect and confidence in the patients comes second to the organizational and economic imperatives. This, he argued, leads to passivity and acceptance of the role of a sick, incapable, dependent patient. His observations and the theory developed from them, especially the processes whereby institutionalization occurs, had a substantial impact on the policies regarding the asylum systems. In part, this contributed to their demise in many parts of the world.

A problem with such generalization is that the researcher is required to make assumptions about what are the essential characteristics of a case or a group and to assume that these are shared in different settings. For example, it might be claimed that at least some hospitals were not organized in this way and Goffman's theory did not apply. However, what many researchers may be doing in such circumstances is to use their clinical knowledge, especially in terms of their experience over many years of working in a variety of contexts. Goffman certainly saw more than one hospital or at least heard, read, and communicated about different settings and the extent to which the processes he described fitted with his broader knowledge.

*What assists such generalizability?*

The following may assist in the process of generalizability of findings:

1 Adequate detail. This involves offering rich details of participants, con-texts, treatments and so on. It allows the readers or consumers of the research to be able to compare and contrast others' findings with their own context.
2 Shared contexts. We can consider and try to map out the extent to which it is possible to assume some shared or dissimilar features between our own and our reader's context. One important aspect of this is that within a culture, for example, we can make some assumptions of similarities: 'the existence of some shared norms, a common language and physical referents can allow at least some . . . viable comparison between places' (Williams, 2000: p. 137).
3 Variation in the context to which we want to generalize our research. The more varied the group to which we are intending to direct our research, the greater the problems of making empirical generalizations from qualitative research. In clinical contexts the populations may be small but can be widely varied. As with quantitative research, if we aim our research at a more homogenous population then we can more legiti-mately make generalizations from qualitative studies, including single-case studies (Gomm *et al.*, 2000).
4 We can make an assumption that our reader has both interest and abilities, such as the use of their imagination, their varied experience of the world and so on, to be able to draw out from our study parts that connect with their own context and experiences (Seale, 1999).
5 Transparency of our own assumptions and the possible selective pro-cesses that may have gone on in the conduct and analysis of our research.
6 We need to be careful, however, that we do not make easy assumptions about similarities within our own culture. If we bear in mind that our readers may have different cultural backgrounds or experiences that can vary within the same culture, this can help us to make these visible in our research. In turn, this can help clarify what aspects are shared and can assist in generalizability even across cultures.

In part, the above points can be seen from a social constructionist stance, which emphasizes the unique local construction of meanings but also emphasizes the power of shared language, symbols, imagery and commen-taries on our shared world. These processes are thought to be iterative, shaped continuously through the media and by our engagement in local conversations that, in turn, are shaped by and reproduce these shared meanings. This means that we have a set of shared referents which helps us to draw out connections and to make generalizations when detailed descriptions are offered of a person's experience in a piece of qualitative research.

For example, in one piece of research the mother of a young woman with a diagnosis of anorexia nervosa described her daughter's experiences of moving from the North of England to a school in the South-west and being teased. It is possible to make connections with such a description, not just on the basis of our personal experience (for example, both of us have experienced moves to alien cultures) but also on the basis of shared themes and stories in our culture. We share some ideas about how Northerners may be different to Southerners and so on. This is not to say these differences are true, but that we know about these common assumptions and that they help us to understand how this mother was also making sense of her experience through some of these shared common assumptions.

## MIXED METHODS: NUMBERS AND MEANINGS

Typically, there has been seen to be a schism between the use of numbers and words in research. But in fact we all use quantification, either formally or informally, to give meaning to events and experiences. For example, when we say, 'Well, I rarely see clients for more than ten sessions', or even if we say, 'The work is going very well', or when a client says, 'I feel a lot better', this involves a quantification. We can then put numbers or categories to such statements to help clarify them, but essentially they contain meanings.

Returning to the example earlier of Goffman's work, we can suggest that almost certainly he was employing informal quantitative ideas – numbers – about how common the sort of processes might be in different hospitals. To develop this as an example, this might have been explored more formally. Thus a variety of hospitals might have been sent questionnaires exploring the extent to which the patients were encouraged to become independent. This might have been directed to both staff and patients. Along with this there could have been measures of how often they engaged in a variety of activities, such as cooking, outings and paid work, whether the work was paid at union rates, the extent of therapy, recourse to medication and so on. This could offer a quantifiable picture of how the institutions were encouraging independence and change as opposed to merely or predominantly 'managing' the patients.

Such data combined with one or more case studies of hospitals, possibly chosen on the basis of being low as opposed to high on the measures of independence, could help contextualize the qualitative findings, perhaps revealing different processes in the different hospital contexts. Interestingly, this is exactly the argument that many institutions levelled as criticism of such studies, 'Ah yes, but it does not represent us.' A combined study can indicate the extent to which the qualitative findings may apply. Probably, it is such evidence that at least partly led to the demise of the asylum, as it was realized that such practices were extremely widespread. Of course, the closures and the move to 'community care' were not simply based on research and therapeutic imperatives but also on economic desires to reduce public spending.

# KEY REFERENCES

Barker, C., Pistrang, N. and Elliott, R. (2002) *Research Methods in Clinical Psychology*, 2nd edn. Chichester: Wiley.

Goffman, E. (1961) *Asylums*. Chicago: Aldine.

Gomm, R., Hammersley, M. and Foster, P. (2000) Case study and generalization, in R. Gomm, M. Hammersley and P. Foster (eds) *Case Study Method*. London: Sage.

Roth. A. and Fonagy, P. (1996) *What Works for Whom?* London: Guilford.

Seale, C. (1999) *The Quality of Qualitative Research*. London: Sage.

Smith, J. A., Osborn, M. and Jarman, M. (1999) Doing interpretative phenomenological analysis, in M. Murray and K. Chamberlain (eds) *Qualitative Health Psychology*. London: Sage.

# 4 ■ CHOOSING A QUALITATIVE METHOD

## CHAPTER OVERVIEW

This chapter offers a guide to choosing between the major approaches to qualitative research. We have decided to offer this because, in our experience as research supervisors, such a guide is not readily available in texts on qualitative research or elsewhere. The chapter outlines some comparisons and contrasts between the different qualitative approaches, along with examples of applications of each of them. We start with an overview of the guiding assumptions which link qualitative research and which distinguish these from quantitative methods. We then consider the approaches which involve analysis of text, for example, from interviews, therapy transcriptions and case study and observational research. Suggestions are offered for the kinds of research questions that each might be best able to address.

Although the approaches are outlined in terms of the procedures involved, this chapter continues the core themes of the book: the clinical relevance of research approaches that emphasise meanings and experience; approaches that promote reflective practice, especially in the interpretative process involved in the analysis of data; approaches that lend themselves to collaborative effort; and designs that are small scale and do-able.

# INTRODUCTION

Qualitative methods of research design are evolving rapidly and gaining credibility within the psychotherapy research field. We are faced with an increasing number of choices about what might be the best approach to the study of our research question and analysis of our data. In the main, we choose a qualitative method if our research question is oriented towards the exploration and understanding of meaning, rather than the direct testing of a concept or hypothesis. Within the psychotherapy field, there are a number of areas of interest that rely on understanding participants' viewpoints, such as user views of the therapy process and outcomes, the meaning of change and models of change in therapy and cross-cultural variations in understanding. Qualitative methods tend to rely on interviews, focus groups and other forms of structured and/or focused interviews, such as the Delphi method or Elliott's method of interpersonal process recall (Elliott, 1984), transcriptions of therapy sessions and observational methods to collect data for analysis. Clearly some methods of data collection, such as observational methods, repertory grids and grounded theory designs lend themselves also to mixed method designs.

Given the increasing range of methods of qualitative research available, there is little in the way of guidance about how to choose between the different approaches. Our aim in this chapter is to offer some pointers to how we might start to think about this choice. We acknowledge at the outset that this is an ambitious task. There are variations within as well as between the approaches and we cannot hope to represent all of the subtle debates and nuances of the methods. However, psychotherapy researchers need a place to start and to have at least some idea of what the different qualitative approaches might contribute. We have attempted to do this by outlining what we see to be some of the key features that distinguish between the approaches and by offering illustrations of their applications. A combination of the two should help when making decisions about what type of analysis to attempt.

## KEY FEATURES

As a starting point we offer a summary of some of the key features of qualitative approaches, though not all of them will share these fully.
Qualitative methods in our view:

- Focus on understanding, for example, the meanings attributed to people's actions and intentions.
- Emphasize rich descriptions of a phenomenon and allow participants' voices to be heard, for example, by providing contextualized verbatim quotes from participants.
- Argue that human experience and behaviour is to be viewed in its context and its full complexity.
- Recognize variability of meanings over time and across contexts.
- Emphasize subjectivity – the recognition of some uniqueness within individual experience and behaviour.
- Use inductive methods of analysis and attempt to generate theory rather than test it.
- Facilitate generalization of findings to existing theory by providing adequate descriptions and evidence for the reader to make connections with their own experience.
- Hold an acknowledged interpretative stance – it is assumed that understanding participants' accounts necessarily involves a process of interpretation.
- Adopt a reflexive stance – interpretation of data is at least partly subjective and shaped by the researcher's own experiences, beliefs and attitudes, which can be made more transparent through dialogue with a research supervisor, keeping a research diary, talking with research participants and through the detail of the audit trail.

Thus when we judge the usefulness of qualitative research, we use a number of criteria to guide us. The research needs to be interesting and accessible to the reader, using tables and illustrations where possible. We want to be drawn into the account and feel involved in thinking about the application of the findings to our practice. We want to hear the participants' 'voices', not just the researcher's account of what people might have to say. We look for the capacity to reflect on the methods used, the interpretation of the findings and the consideration of alternatives, along with reflections on the researcher's own stance and their biases and how they influenced the research process. Has the researcher explored the context of the research for its impact on the conduct of the research and the interpretation of the findings? To what extent have the participants been involved in a collaborative design?

There are some key differences between the qualitative designs, largely based in their philosophical wellsprings. The different social science traditions have given rise to different methods of qualitative design and data analysis, sometimes used in unidisciplinary isolation. The psycho-therapy field offers a unique site for collaboration and comparative analysis of the suitability of the various methods for our purposes as psychotherapists. For example, the humanistic field has given rise to action research and cooperative enquiry, favoured by educational psychology and counselling for approaching local workplace-related questions. The traditions of phenomenology, symbolic interactionism and constructivism have given us grounded theory and its variants (originally developed in sociology), theme analysis, interpretative phenomenological analysis and the anthropological methods of ethnography. Social constructionism and symbolic interactionism have influenced literary and linguistic methods of analysis, such as narrative analysis, rhetorical analysis, conversation analysis and discourse analysis, and have found their place in social psychology, sociology and the systemic field. This variety gives rise to differences in the kinds of questions these methods might address, the underlying conceptual assumptions and the type of data that might be generated.

We are pragmatic in our approach to research design and find that some of the methods can be combined in ways that best address our questions, as long as we remain clear about their philosophical differences and the implications of any combination! A core issue for us is that, whatever combination of research methods and analyses we choose to employ, we make sure we provide sufficiently detailed evidence from our participants to substantiate our analysis. In this way, we can be sure our methods of analysis and our reporting of the data are culturally sensitive. We would suggest that it is in our interpretation of how qualitative methods should be used that risks of ethnocentrism lie (implicit assumptions based upon our cultural attitudes and prejudices), rather than with the methods themselves. Additional ethnographic strategies can always be used to further contextualize the data. Cultural sensitivity within our own culture can be enhanced, for example, by emphasizing a collaborative research approach whereby we incorporate clients' views and participation in the research from the outset. Equally, we may recruit other colleagues or clients of different culture, gender or ethnicity to help offer a broader range of interpretations of our data. For us, the real challenge posed by qualitative methods is found in the demands made on us as psychotherapy researchers to perceive sensitively and to conceptualize the complexity within the data, in a way in which the findings are both grounded in the material and culturally attuned. We see this as the main bridge between our clinical practice and our psychotherapy research practice.

Unlike quantitative research design, most of the qualitative research methods do not manualize the method of analysis using step-by-step approaches. This can be daunting for the novice researcher. In the following section, we look briefly at some of the major approaches to qualitative analysis and, where possible draw lessons from our own experience of using the methods to help you choose amongst them. We will then outline and draw comparisons between the following: grounded theory; interpretative phenomenological analysis; discourse analysis and rhetorical analysis; narrative analysis; and qualitative observation.

## WHICH METHOD SHOULD I CHOOSE?

We have broadly grouped the qualitative methods into the following five categories. This is a simplification and many would argue that there are many more that could be included. However, these are the most widely applied approaches and have been employed to some extent in counselling and psychotherapy research studies.

| | |
|---|---|
| **Interpretative theme analyses** | These approaches broadly start from the premise that people have relatively stable ways of viewing their experiences and the task of research is to get as close to these beliefs, schemas, cognitions, themes as we possibly can. In order to do this an interpretative process on the part of the researcher is required. This is a constructivist view which argues that there are external realities but we can only ever know them through our own subjective lenses. |
| **Discourse analysis** | This starts from the premise that human experience is constructed in interactions, predominantly in conversations between people. People's understandings, explanations, ideas and so on are not seen as necessarily enduring but as more immediately constructed in various situations according to whom they are interacting with. Central to this construction is the use of language. |
| **Narrative analysis** | These approaches are concerned to explore the stories that people hold about their lives and how our sense of self and identity is shaped by the stories that we hold. The emphasis is on events over time, that stories connect up the past, present and the future. The emphasis is on the personal accounts that people hold. Also, stories and narratives are explored in terms of their power to evoke feelings and how they offer a coherence or sense of purpose to the person's life. |
| **Qualitative observation** | These approaches are interested in exploring phenomena by engaging in observations. These may be at various levels of involvement but recognize that observation is also an interpretative process. They make use of the researcher's reflections on their feelings, beliefs and expectations in situations under study. |
| **Case study** | These studies attempt a detailed and holistic analysis in an attempt to capture the clinical phenomena in its full complexity. There is a close resemblance between a thorough clinical case study and a research case study. The research can employ a variety of forms of data, such as observation, interviews, analysis of clinical sessions, life history and case notes, and a variety of people may contribute to the case study, such as family members, therapist, client's observations and the researcher's own reflections. The studies often extend over time, allowing a longitudinal analysis of how events unfold and change occurs. |

# INTERPRETATIVE THEME ANALYSES

There are a number of reasons for choosing an interpretative theme analysis:

- The researcher wants to understand and represent the participants' point of view, perhaps adopting a critical realist position in relation to knowledge.
- The researcher assumes that the participants' point of view, in terms of constructs and assumptions, is relatively stable over time.
- The researcher wants to extract major themes and issues in participants' accounts.
- The researcher wants to develop hypotheses and small-scale theories that connect the themes.

There are two main types of interpretative theme analysis: grounded theory and interpretative phenomenological analysis (IPA). One of the key differences is that grounded theory makes more ambitious claims to develop formal (generalizable to a broader population) theory from the studies, whereas IPA is content to offer a more descriptive and local theory. We will offer a description of both approaches in part, since grounded theory also lays some of the conceptual ground for interpretative approaches such as IPA. Both approaches typically rely on interviews in order to generate accounts from participants about areas of experience. In addition, both typically involve small group studies, the intention of which is to emerge with themes that are common to the participants and carry the salient features of their experience.

## Grounded theory

The basis of grounded theory is the idea that any theory gains meaning by being grounded in good, powerful, convincing examples. Though characteristically associated with qualitative research it also applies to quantitative research, in that for a theory to have any meaning we need to see examples of what it means. Hence this is a general concept for qualitative research. Nevertheless, the approaches differ in the extent to which they attempt to develop formal theory or are content to let evidence – for example, participants' accounts, or participant researchers' observations speak for themselves. The idea of 'grounding theory' was developed by Glaser and Strauss during the 1960s at the Chicago School of Sociology into an approach termed 'grounded theory'. Since that time it has been developed for use in different countries, with different disciplines and for different research questions.

A common strand is a wish to discover theory in the systematic collection and analysis of data using inductive as opposed to deductive methods. This stems from Glaser and Strauss' (1967) original critique of the hypothetico-deductive method of theory testing and their attempt to broaden our view of how social scientists might approach research. Such research can be seen as empirical studies or problem solving approaches that seek to understand action from the perspective of the human agent. The aim is to generate middle range theories to help understand human experience and phenomena.

## Grounded theory studies

There are a number of reasons for choosing grounded theory:

- The researcher wants to develop middle range theories that help explain an under-theorized area of human experience.
- The researcher wants to stay close to the data and perform a detailed analysis of the text.
- The researcher wants to use a method of analysis that keeps their own interpretative activity at bay until later stages of the analysis.
- The researcher wants to develop progressive hypotheses and small-scale theories using methods of theoretical sampling, constant comparison, axial coding and memo writing.
- The researcher wants to delay the literature review until their own research hypotheses begin to develop.
- The researcher wants to continue sampling until theoretical saturation is achieved.

An example of a grounded theory study is given in Research Example 4.1.

### Research Example 4.1

Helmeke, K. and Sprenkle, D. (2000) Clients' perceptions of pivotal moments in couples therapy: a qualitative study of change in therapy, *Journal of Marital and Family Therapy*, 26: 469–83.

The authors wanted to study change process in couples therapy from the point of view of the clients. They collected data from three sources: analysis of therapy session transcripts; post-session questionnaires; and two post-therapy interviews with three white, heterosexual couples. The three sources of data were analysed as the research proceeded. Thus the analysis fostered the development of formative theory and further guided data collection.

The data analysis consisted of careful initial coding of the data and employed the method of constant comparison, whereby emerging themes are systematically compared and contrasted in order to produce the most convincing themes. This process continues until there is a 'saturation' so that the analysis of further data produces no new themes. An important step in this process is to deliberately attempt to find cases that might produce differences.

From the analysis it was discovered that a key theme was that of 'pivotal moments'. The participants identified specific therapy events or moments as pivotal. These pivotal moments were highly individualized accounts, and interestingly, with little overlap between spouses and with little overlap between clients' and therapists' identification of pivotal moments. These were seen to occur during discussions of problems areas for the spouses and after repeated discussions of the same topic. The authors suggest that these pivotal moments can be conceptualized as small outcomes within each session. They also found a theme of different experiences in that within a piece of couple's therapy there appeared to be three therapy processes: her therapy; his therapy; and the therapist's therapy. The findings were seen to add to psychotherapy process theory.

### Description of the method

The approach uses structured methods to collect and analyse the data. Typically this involves interviews, although other sources of materials, as above, may be employed. A central feature is that of theoretical sampling so that cases for inclusion in the study are selected on a progressive basis to test and extend the emerging theory. This typically means that data collection and analysis proceed simultaneously. The researcher does not start with a preconceived hypothesis; rather the early data analysis drives the development of hypotheses and subsequent data gathering. The initial literature review supports the development of the research question, identifies the question as sitting within an under-theorized area, but does not proceed further at this stage. The main literature review is delayed until analysis is well under way, and is driven by the emergent findings. Such an approach to literature reviewing in the field of psychotherapy can encourage seeking literature in other psychotherapy fields and other social science disciplines, which enriches our understandings and encourages cross-discipline 'talking'!

### Stages in the analysis

1 The analysis attempts to create analytic codes and categories from the data that reflect the interaction between the researcher and participant and that shape subsequent data collection. The interview or observation transcripts are coded, using a process called 'line by line' coding. This can be a line of text, a meaningful grammatical phrase or a sentence (it is useful to double space the transcript and leave wide margins for writing the initial codes).

2 Alongside this coding, the researcher notes their own reflections – thoughts, emotional reactions and connections to theory – as separate 'memos', which are returned to later in the analysis. Unlike IPA which incorporates the researcher's interpretative stance at the start of the data analysis procedures, grounded theory methods seek to get alongside what is being said and limit inferential interpretation of the data as much as is possible at this stage.

In creating these line by line codes and summarizing the meaning expressed in the text, Charmaz (1995) recommends asking the following questions:

- What is going on in the data?
- What are people doing?
- What do these actions and statements take for granted?
- How do structure and context serve to support, maintain, impede or change these actions and statements?

Thus Charmaz recommends looking at action in relation to meaning. For example, what are the explanations for action offered, what are the unstated assumptions about it, what are the intentions for engaging in action, what are the effects on others, and what are the consequences for interpersonal relationships and for further action?

3 Once the first transcript has been coded these can be combined into a first-level category analysis using a process of focused coding. These categories identify the collective properties of the codes and may well be grouped together in terms of their contextual features, such as where and when they occur, the consequences of the action in the categories, what maintains the action and so on. In our experience, it is easy to become lost in the many line by line codes that can be developed from one transcript. Computer programs, such as NUDIST, are available to assist in this analysis but unless large numbers of interviews or data are involved it may be more meaningful to stay physically close to the data. Part of the reflective process may be to ask questions, such as: what is at issue here? How does the research participant think, feel and act? What is happening? What is changing? What are the effects of what is happening?

4 Once the codes from the first transcript have been organized into categories the relationship between the categories can be explored; this is constant comparison. At this point the study can move to recruiting the next participant. The selection is based on what theory has started to emerge from the initial analysis. So, for example, if you were conducting an exploratory study into vegetarianism, and why people choose to become vegetarians, and your first analysis suggested a slow considered process of decision making, you might be curious to know if other approaches to decision making had been used. The act of trying to identify similarities and differences in the categories engages us in a process of hypothesizing, and then progressive hypothesizing as we move iteratively through the analysis of further transcripts, much as in the way we employ the process of hypothesizing in our clinical work. The hypotheses we develop help us to explain behaviour and processes at work in the data. Grounded theorists continue the process of sampling and analysis until the point of saturation, that is, when further sampling and analysis of data does not add further to the developing understanding and explanation.

5 Memo-writing proceeds alongside the early analytic process. It is a way of recording our reactions to the analytic method and to the data. We may find ourselves making early comparisons, drawing on extant theory, wondering about latent motivations and seeking relationships between beliefs, actions, events and people. This activity informs theoretical sampling, that is, going back and sampling for the purpose of developing our emerging hypotheses into middle range theory. Since memo-writing promotes a self-reflexive analysis of the processes and assumptions that

underpin the development of our codes and categories, it helps explicate our thinking during the process of constant comparison, where we seek similarities and differences between our categories.

Thus grounded theory methods try to delay inference and interpretation, as much as possible, until later on in the process of analysis. The final stage of our literature review begins as we compare how our findings sit within the extant literature, and further develop thinking in our chosen area of enquiry.

## Interpretative phenomenological analysis

There are a number of reasons for choosing interpretative phenomeno-logical analysis:

- The researcher wants to understand the points of view of the participants and represent them as main issues and themes.
- The researcher wants to use their own interpretative activity to help them understand and interpret the participants' points of view at the beginning of the analytic process.
- The researcher wants to compare themes across two groups of participants.
- The researcher is less interested in modelling the themes and issues, and more interested in connecting the themes to existing literature.
- The researcher is conducting a small-scale study with a small sample size and cannot engage in the process of theoretical sampling.

An example of an IPA study is given in Research Example 4.2.

---

**Research Example 4.2**

Osborn, M. and Smith, J. (1998) The personal experience of chronic benign lower back pain: an interpretative phenomenological analysis, *British Journal of Health Psychology*, 3: 65–83.

Chronic lower back pain is a major health problem and one where pain, physical impairment and biological pathology are only very loosely correlated. It is considered that the experience of pain, its distress and disability is mediated by its meaning to the sufferer. The intention of this study was to explore the sufferer's personal experience of their pain. Semi-structured interviews were carried out on a small sample of nine women suffering with chronic back pain. The verbatim transcripts of those interviews served as data for an IPA analysis. The transcripts were analysed for initial concepts or codes. The researchers held some tentative preliminary theory that changes in identity might emerge as an important theme. Reflective notes were kept to enable the researcher both to employ and also to be able to remain sensitive to other important themes that might emerge. Four themes emerged which were described under the broad headings: searching for an explanation; comparing this self with other selves; not being believed; and withdrawing from others.

The participants shared an inability to explain the persistent presence of their pain or to reconstruct any contemporary self-regard. While they used social comparison to try to help them make sense of their situation, these comparisons proved equivocal in their outcome. They described how they were unable to establish the legitimacy of the chronic nature of their pain and in certain situations felt obliged to appear ill to conform to the expectations of others. By default, participants treated their own pain as a stigma and tended to withdraw from social contact. They felt confused, afraid for their future and vulnerable to shame.

### Description of the method

Interpretative phenomenological analysis (Smith, 1996; Smith et al., 1999; Reid et al., 2005) has found recent popularity in psychology and psychotherapy research, particularly amongst health practitioners. Here the emphasis is on people's abilities to reflect on and give meanings to their lives. The approach is phenomenological in its focus on how individuals make sense of events or experiences associated with the topic under study. The approach is constructionist in its assumption that meaning is generated through interpretative processes, for both the participant and the researcher. Language and context are believed to shape a person's responses to his or her understanding of events or personal experiences. People are assumed to be capable of consciously reflecting on most aspects of their lives.

We can draw a distinction here with some of the discursive methods, that seek to use psychoanalytic theory to understand latent processes in the text, or the defences that we use to rhetorically position ourselves in relation to the topic under study. IPA assumes that people hold relatively stable cognitions, beliefs or schemas that can be accessed readily through interview or other methods, such as focus groups or open-ended questionnaires. The role of the researcher is to try to get as near as possible to these cognitions or schemas by carefully analysing accounts using an ideographic approach. The detailed analysis of small numbers of participants' interviews can lead to cautious generalization to existing theory. The approach is interpretative because it involves a process of interpretation on the part of the researcher. The researcher's inferences, biases and reactions are made evident (as far as this is possible) and actively recruited into the analytic process at a very early stage of the analysis.

The methodology of an IPA study combines purposive sampling with flexible use of open-ended questions in semi-structured interview schedules. Typically, small group designs are employed using semi-structured interviews with individuals representative of an area of experience, for example, young offenders' accounts of their violent behaviour, women's experience of chronic back pain or children's experience of another child being adopted into their family. IPA designs are usually cross-sectional with a one-off interview offering a picture of how the group of participants view their experience at a particular point in time. The findings from two small groups can be used in an exploratory comparative study. Each participant or transcript can be treated in its own right as a case study, with each analysis contributing to the case study series. Analysis can be started once the interviews are completed, but the grounded theory methods of constant comparison and theoretical sampling can be imported to adapt the IPA to suit a more ethnographic approach to hypothesis development.

## The analysis process

IPA analysis proceeds in a stepwise manner:

1 Each transcript is read in detail a few times.
2 The search for themes begins with a two-margin approach to coding. Use the left-hand margin to identify key words and phrases, or to summarize the meaning in a small chunk of text. The detailed approach of line by line coding is not used. The researcher determines the size of the 'chunk': it may be a phrase or it may be a paragraph. When coding in the left-hand margin, identify the speaker attached to the code, for subsequent analysis of similarities and differences in the themes identified for each speaker.
3 Use the right margin to annotate your inferences, assumptions and reactions to the text, especially any connections made with existing theory. This two-margin approach to initial coding of the transcript can be contrasted to the search for micro-linguistic structures and features found in conversation analysis.
4 Once the whole transcript has been coded using the two-margin approach, list all the left-hand codes chronologically and search for connections between the codes. Cluster the codes according to existing theory and your clinical experience. This process of clustering relies on the analytic and interpretative process of the researcher, driven by the right-hand margin comments.
5 Next, give the clustered codes a category title – these become the emergent themes. Additionally, in the right-hand margin inferences can be clustered separately to help the researcher make explicit their biases and assumptions, and their use of implicit theory, in the service of a self-reflexive analysis. Understanding how our assumptions both explicitly drive and potentially covertly influence our approach to data sampling, analysis and interpretation is crucial to an IPA study. However, the IPA approach does not explicitly theorize self-reflexivity as a process. We have found that encouraging research students to theme analyse their right-hand margin comments along with their research diary notes identifies key issues and themes that help the reader interpret the findings and make judgements about their trustworthiness. These self-reflexive themes can also be subjected to the methods of constant comparison, and reflexive hypotheses can be developed.
6 The emergent themes can be clustered into superordinate themes, and if desired, clustered again, into master level themes. Each category level can

be named using the interpretative commentary found in the right-hand margin notes. The decision as to how far to take the category analysis of themes is often determined by the level of abstraction required. Clearly, each stage of clustering strips meaning from the text and risks taking us further away from what was being said in the original transcript. We always encourage our research students to use full and descriptive names for their new categories or themes. Each level of theme analysis should be grounded in the text, and it should be possible to find direct quotations to support the theme analysis. This is the audit trail.

The IPA analysis can be conducted in full on each transcript in the study, whilst recognizing that each subsequent IPA analysis will be influenced by the previous one. Then the superordinate themes or master themes (depending at which level the researcher closes the theme analysis) can be pooled to represent common themes in the study. Alternatively, using the grounded theory method of constant comparison, the superordinate or master level themes from each transcript in the study can be compared and contrasted, facilitating a process of hypothesis development or of psychological modelling. Another alternative is to develop a short cut approach with a larger number of qualitative interview transcripts. A full IPA analysis can be conducted on three or four studies in the bottom-up inductive manner. The IPA master themes can be pooled across these studies, and then the pooled categories can be used to read subsequent transcripts, in a 'top-down' manner. Direct quotations are sought to support such a 'top-down' reading. In addition, new themes are spotted where they occur. Either way, the process of IPA analysis is iterative and re-labelling of themes with subsequent analysis is likely to occur.

The results of an IPA study are usually presented as themes that are held in common by members of the group. Themes can be presented in tabular format, showing the clustering and sub-clustering of themes, supported by direct quotations. Sometimes there is an emphasis on identifying a limited number of core or central themes, or sometimes in representing all the themes. The nature of an IPA theme is flexible. For example, it can be a specific topic under question, a more general sense of a person's beliefs or style of thinking or an overarching category that makes sense of all the material. In addition, the themes can be presented as a case study series, comparing and contrasting the themes across each participant, or as a small group comparison. The themes can be turned into a narrative account, whereby the discussion centres on how the themes are grounded in the transcripts. Caution is needed when generalizing themes to theory and to implications for clinical practice. Validity is usually approached through the audit trail, with respondent validation or with the help of independent auditors as to whether the arguments developed are warranted in the light of the data (see Chapter 10 for further discussion).

IPA has a broadly similar inductive, bottom-up approach to data analysis as found in grounded theory. It also shares a similar epistemological base to grounded theory. In our view, IPA is a very rigorous and systematic approach to interpretative theme analysis. It is grounded in psychological thinking and uses extant theory early on in the analytic process, whereas grounded theory attempts to delay the process of inference and stick closer to the detail of the participants' talk. The IPA themes can be represented as a list of key issues and themes that can inform service planning and delivery, for example, with service user feedback. By importing grounded theory methods of constant comparison and theoretical sampling, hypotheses can be developed to link the IPA themes and these themes can be used to model putative psychological processes. IPA sits within the grounded methods of qualitative analysis in our view, rather than within the more discursive methods, because it is interested in people's attitudes and cognitions rather than in the language used by participants to rhetorically position themselves in relation to the topic under study.

Research Example 4.3 outlines an IPA study in a clinical context:

---

**Research Example 4.3**

Crouch, W. and Wright, J. (2004) A qualitative investigation into deliberate self-harm at an adolescent mental health unit, *Clinical Child Psychology and Psychiatry*, in press.

Deliberate self-harm is a serious problem for significant numbers of adolescents. It has been shown to be especially prevalent in institutions like mental health units where 'contagion' of the behaviour has been observed to occur. This investigation aimed to identify the personal and interpersonal processes involved in deliberate self-harm at a residential treatment setting for adolescents with mental health problems. Interviews and participant observation were used. Six adolescents on the unit with a history of deliberate self-harm were interviewed about their perceptions of deliberate self-harm. Process notes taken at the unit 'community meeting' were used to provide support for the themes generated in the interviews.

The interviews were analysed using interpretative phenomenological analysis. Deliberate self-harm seemed to be in response to conflict or feeling upset or angry. It could make those around the adolescent harming themselves feel angry, upset and burdened by feeling they should respond. Subgroups of 'self-harming for genuine reasons' and 'self-harming for attention' emerged as a central theme. Adolescents seemed to compete to be the 'most genuine' self-harmer. This could cause them to feel they needed to cause a certain level of damage when self-harming and to harm themselves in secret. Seeking help appeared difficult.

It was concluded that group treatment methods were indicated, as well as challenging the traditional response to deliberate self-harm of not giving attention. Further research seemed crucial and some ideas for this are outlined.

---

## Theme analysis

It is worth mentioning a simpler form of theme analysis at this point in the discussion. Often, when developing and honing our research question, we may conduct preliminary or pilot investigations that generate unstructured data. Theme analysis is used to order such data. Typically we read the data sources a few times first, then jot down issues of interest, ideas, repetition and key words and phrases that we see in the data. Then we list these themes on a separate sheet and search for clusters or connections. Some of the themes will follow from our pilot enquiry, while some may be new. We may ask of each person we pilot our research question with, what are three important things I have learned from this person, or about this person? These themes can then be used to inform the development of the research question. Although this is a 'quick and dirty' method that does not engage directly with issues of reflexivity, it often reveals key issues and helps confirm or disconfirm the proposed direction of our research.

An example of theme analysis is outlined in Research Example 4.4.

---

**Research Example 4.4**

Woodward, C. and Joseph, S. (2003) Positive change processes and post-traumatic growth in people who have experienced childhood abuse: understanding vehicles of change, *Psychology and Psychotherapy-Theory Research and Practice*, 76: 267–83.

Post-traumatic growth is an emerging area of research concerned with the positive psychological changes that can follow the experience of traumatic events. The aim of this study was to explore themes of post-traumatic growth within personal experience narratives of individuals who have experienced some form of early emotional, physical or sexual abuse. Using thematic analysis, three domains of themes were identified that related to positive change processes: inner drive towards growth; vehicles of change; and psychological changes. Understanding the different vehicles of change has implications for facilitating post-traumatic growth in clients who have experienced traumatic events.

---

## THE DISCURSIVE METHODS

There are a number of reasons for choosing discursive methods

- The researcher adopts a social constructionist position and assumes that language is constitutive and constructive.
- The researcher is interested in all forms of talk and text.
- Discourse is believed to be central to the negotiation of our shared social realities, in which we use discourse to *do* things, such as blame, apologize, present ourselves in a positive light and so on.
- The researcher wants to approach the text with a higher level of inference.
- The researcher may wish to undertake a theoretical reading of the text.
- The reading of the text produced belongs to the researcher and they have responsibility for warranting their particular reading.

## Discourse analysis

There are a number of reasons for choosing discourse analysis:

- The researcher wants to explore the construction of meaning in social relationships.
- Discourses are believed to reflect power relations and are thus subject to change over time and in different social and cultural contexts. Thus researchers want to explore how social and cultural trends and contexts show up in text.
- The researcher seeks to understand how specific discourses are undermined or promoted.
- The researcher wants to analyse what is hidden or buried within the text, the so-called subtext, as well as what is overtly discussed within the text.

An example of discourse analysis is given in Research Example 4.5.

**Research Example 4.5**

Frosh, S., Phoenix, A., and Pattman, R. (2000) 'But it's racism I really hate': Young masculinities, racism, and psychoanalysis, *Psychoanalytic Psychology*, 17(2): 225–42.

This article addresses the issue of how discursive analyses can reveal the way personal accounts of masculinities are constructed and can be supplemented by theories providing plausible explanations of how individuals take up particular subject positions. It is suggested that psychoanalytic concepts are helpful in this regard. An analysis is presented of material from a participant in a study of emergent masculinities among boys in London schools. This material concerns the cross-cutting of gendered and racialized identity positions. The use of psychoanalytic constructs enables the production of an account of this participant's narrative in which reasons for his adoption and defence of particular positions, despite their contradictory and conflictual character, can be proposed.

### Description of the method

Wetherell *et al.* (2001) have identified at least six different approaches to discourse analysis. The discursive methods have arisen out of the relationship between literary analysis of texts and the social constructionist movement within psychology and psychotherapy. Broadly speaking, these approaches share a view that knowledge about ourselves and about others is culturally bounded, and that different cultural systems entail different psychologies, which reflexively influence the social sciences (Gill, 1996). The different perspectives that make up 'discourse analysis' do not assume that language simply describes or reflects social reality. Rather they assume that language, and hence discourse, is central to the negotiation of our shared social realities. People are thought to struggle in their use of language over the nature of events.

Discourse is a somewhat elusive term. We define it pragmatically in terms of all forms of talk and text, whether they be interview transcripts, published text or naturally occurring conversation. Discourses are seen to be the constructs, often derived from wider social and cultural repertoires, which individuals use to present accounts of their actions and experiences. Some discourses are believed to be more dominant in our society than in others and to change over time.

In general terms, we can describe discourse analysts as being interested in talk and texts in terms of their content and organization. Discursive analysis is underpinned by the belief that language is constitutive and constructive, that is, that discourse is manufactured out of existing linguistic resources and that talk and texts construct our world, in that we do not deal with our world in direct, unmediated ways. This notion of construction as metaphor implies that in the development of any account, there is choice – choice amongst alternative descriptions – and that any choice depends upon the orientation of the speaker or writer. Discourse analysts are concerned with the action or function orientation of the talk and text under scrutiny.

Discourse is considered to be a social practice, in that people use discourse to *do* things, such as to blame others, to self-justify, to persuade, to apologize or make excuses, to take or evade responsibility for actions and to show up in a positive light. This assumes that discourse does not take place in a social and cultural vacuum. Our version of events could well depend on who we were talking to at the time! Thus discourse analysts are interested in both the interpretative context and the interpretative repertoires of both participants and researchers. Discourse is treated as being organized rhetorically, with the assumption that much discourse is involved in establishing one view of the world in the face of competing or marginalized versions. Advertising and party politics provide strong examples of how rhetoric is used to persuade us to adopt one point of view over another.

Discursive studies focus on how participants construct accounts to explain and justify their actions. For example, there have been studies of how sexual offenders explain their actions and how psychiatrists make decisions about the diagnosis of psychosis. Discourse analysis attempts an analysis not just of what is overtly being discussed but also of what is underlying or hidden – the so-called subtexts. In this way discourse analysis bears some connections with a psychodynamic analysis. In fact many discourse analysts have a strong affinity with psychodynamic theory (Hollway, 1989). Discourse analysis does not assume that there are fundamental beliefs, cognitions or schemas in people's heads but that meanings are constructed in social relationships. In this sense the research interview is itself an example of social construction and attempts are made to subject it to an analysis.

One version of discourse analysis focuses on how dominant discourses (constellations of ideas) are internalized and used to make sense of ourselves and others. The analysis looks for examples of these in people's accounts, such as how dominant ideas of mental health, gender roles or family life shape our ideas (Stenner, 1993). Discourse analysis relies on an awareness of the social, political and cultural trends and contexts to which our texts refer. For example, Hollway (1989) argues that heterosexual couple talk is held in place by 'male sex drive', 'have/hold' and 'permissive' discourses. Doing a discourse analysis means we have to find a way of making analytical sense of texts in all their fragmented, contradictory messiness.

Discourse analysts do not tend to write descriptions of how they conduct the analysis, thus we shall attempt to delineate a few guidelines here. They ask particular questions about the language used in a text:

- What actions does this piece of talk perform?
- What accounts are individuals trying to construct in interaction with each other?
- How do these accounts change as contexts change?
- What are the limitations and consequences of the discourses that individuals use?

### Steps in the analysis

1 Analysis begins with repeat readings of the text – the process of 'immersion' in the data. Prior to analysis questions of interest have been identified, but the method is sufficiently flexible to allow for alteration as the reading progresses.
2 The text can be 'interrogated' from a number of theoretical viewpoints. Alternative readings are encouraged. For example, how might the reading be different from someone of the opposite gender, of a different age or of a different ethnicity? This facilitates suspension of belief in what might normally be taken for granted in language use as well as a shift to the ways in which accounts are constructed.
3 Analysis often has two phases: the function orientation of the text, and the search for pattern in the text. For example, how is the writer attempting to portray him or herself? What rhetorical strategies are being used to persuade, explain, problem solve and so on? Search for pattern and themes in the data, and for consistencies and inconsistencies. Focus on depth and submerged meanings: what appear to be underlying implicit meanings?

The design of discourse analysis studies typically involves interviewing a group of people who share some common features of interest, for example sexual offenders (Gilgun, 1995). Interest is often triggered by questions in terms of how such a group explains, makes sense of or justifies their actions.

## Rhetorical analysis

There are a number of reasons for choosing rhetorical analysis:

- The researcher is interested in how people struggle in their language over the nature of events.

- The researcher is interested in conversation as argument, justification and criticism and how people position themselves and others.
- Rhetorical analysis focuses on issues of accountability and agency in talk.

An example of rhetorical analysis is given in Research Example 4.6.

---

**Research Example 4.6**

Auburn, T. and Lea, S. (2003) Doing cognitive distortions: a discursive psychology analysis of sex offender treatment talk, *British Journal of Social Psychology*, 42: 281–98.

Theories of sex offending have for several years relied upon the notion of cognitive distortions as an important cause of sexual offending. In this study the authors critique this notion and suggest that the sort of phenomenon addressed by cognitive distortions is better understood by adopting a discursive psychology approach. In their approach talk is regarded as occasioned and action oriented. Thus 'cognitive distortions' are conceptualized as something people do rather than something that people have.

Sessions from a prison-based sex offender treatment programme were taped and transcribed. A discursive psychology analysis was conducted on those sessions relating to offenders' first accounts of their offences. The authors' analysis suggests that offenders utilize a particular narrative organization to manage their blame and responsibility for the offence. This organization is based on a first part that is oriented to quotidian precursors to the offence and an immediately following second part that is oriented to a sudden shift in the definition of the situation. The implications of this analysis are discussed, in relation to the status of cognitive distortions and treatment.

---

This is one example of a discursive method. It focuses on action in the text, rather than cognition per se. It views conversation as argument, justification and criticism and focuses on issues of accountability and agency. Stancombe and White (1997) describe a range of rhetorical strategies that we all might use in presenting one version of events, or one view of the world, in order to persuade the other. These include:

- Unhappy incidents – presentation of events as happening due to chance.
- Use of 'facts' – this can have a rhetorical purpose to persuade or justify, to assign accountability, to invite confirmation or to disguise or disown our 'stake' in the matter.
- Extreme case formulation – to present our case in an extreme, exaggerated way in order to increase the impact of our point of view.
- Use of vagueness – this strategy avoids refutation, or at least makes it harder!
- Category entitlement – supporting our account by emphasizing that we belong to a prestigious group.

- Use of common-sense maxims – employing the idea that what we are saying is clear 'common sense'.

When using a rhetorical analysis approach to text, we can ask the following questions: How do the identified discourses position the speaker in the interaction, and/or how does the speaker position him or herself in relation to the discourses? How are specific discourses (interpretative repertoires) promoted or undermined? How are issues of blame and responsibility dealt with? What alternative versions are being constructed in the text? How are challenges to discursive positioning managed? The results of discourse analysis studies are usually presented in terms of characteristic 'rhetorical strategies' or ways of attempting to explain and justify actions. There might be some discussion of inconsistencies, contradictions and defences in people's accounts.

Discourse analysts break with the tradition of treating talk and text as authentic. They impose meanings on another's text. It is not a theory-free approach and, as we indicate above, many analysts use psychoanalytic readings in a 'top-down' analysis of text. This points up some issues of morality and power in research. Whose reading is it? Reflexivity is important. For example, it is important for the researcher to ask why he or she is reading this text in this way. Our own discourse as discourse analysts is no less constructed, occasioned and action oriented than the discourse we are studying! The method of analysis employed profoundly influences the reading and subsequent data collection.

Burman and Parker (1993) identify a number of problems with the practice of discourse analysis. These include: a tendency towards reification in the analysis; the ways in which an analysis can presuppose what it pretends to discover; the use of common-sense knowledge in the elaboration of the categories that are eventually discovered; the treatment of language as more powerful than other material constraints on action; more variability that in human experience and action than is expressed through language; the fact it is a very labour intensive approach; that if we do not know what a text is referring to, we cannot produce a reading; the fact that researchers have responsibility for how their reading will function; the wholesale application of the approach to everything; and the fact it is not a methodology that can be applied to the text without reflecting on the effects of the analysis.

Discourse analysis has identified ways in which relations of domination and subordination are reproduced and justified. Power can be said to be at work in the structural position of people when they are speaking and not speaking. The analysis does not seek general laws or to generalize to a population. Rather it seeks to illuminate the ways in which discourse is constructed from interpretative resources and repertoires in particular interpretative contexts, for example, the way an account is constructed, the kinds of rhetorical resources used and the functions they serve. For these reasons we encourage our students to try to work with colleagues as co-researchers. This helps us note the different ways in which the text could be described, together with other people, in a process of 'free association' to the text.

## NARRATIVE ANALYSIS

There are a number of reasons for choosing narrative analysis:

- The researcher is interested in how people give meanings to their lives in terms of stories or accounts.
- These stories are assumed both to connect events in peoples' lives and explain changes over time.
- Narratives are assumed to have both content and form.
- Feelings and experiences – stories are evocative and we are interested in the feelings that they arouse for the person, and for us, as they talk about their life.

An example of narrative analysis is given in Research Example 4.7.

---

**Research Example 4.7**

Dallos, R., Neale, A. and Strouthos, M. (1997) Pathways to problems: the evolution of 'pathology', *Journal of Family Therapy*, 19(4): 369–401.

This paper describes a qualitative research study that compared accounts from interviews with families where difficulties had evolved into serious problems with those where an escalation of pathology had been avoided. The stories of ten families, each with a young adult member currently experiencing problems and with a serious psychiatric history, were compared with those of eight adults who had no significant current problems and no known psychiatric history.

The accounts of both groups of families were surprisingly similar in details of early distresses and problems. Furthermore, the accounts indicated that family life was commonly seen to be problematic and stressful, particularly during key transitional stages. Specifically, the analysis indicated that it was not simply the severity of the initial stresses and problems that distinguished families, but the meanings that these evoked and the corresponding pattern of responses, especially the 'attempted solutions' that were set in motion. It appeared that these responses, fuelled by negative external interventions, could launch families along pathological pathways. The findings were taken to suggest that the meanings ascribed to difficulties and the ensuing responses were predominantly shaped and constrained by three factors: the dominant socially shared discourses of mental health and distress; the emotional resources and attachments of family members; and systemic and interpersonal processes.

---

*Description of the method*

Narrative analysis emphasizes the idea that people give meanings to their lives through stories that connect events over time and that offer an unfolding and developing picture of their lives. The emphasis is on changes in participants' lives and how each change is given sense by the person in terms of previous events and other transitions. The assumption is that narratives have both content and form:

1 *Content.* How specific events are described and meanings ascribed to them, such as how a loss may have given someone a new sense of meaning and urgency about getting on with important aspects of their life. (See Seltzer and Seltzer, 2004, for an example.)
2 *Form.* The nature of narratives in terms of how coherent they are, how detailed or sparse, how consistently events are connected causally and whether there is a sense of development in the narrative – a sense of purpose, adding up to something, or a 'point' to the story.

There are various forms of narrative research, but they share a focus on facilitating the participants to tell their own stories in their own ways. Hence the interview questions may be very broad, and in autobiographical interviews we can start with one general invitation for the person to talk about their life. Related to this, further interview questions are intended to help the person to articulate more details or give examples (such as episodes) of particular parts of their story rather than to steer their story in a different direction. In narrative research the order in which people present the events in their life is important because it can reveal that apparently relatively minor events can hold significance for them and that their story may not be chronologically ordered. Sometimes we remember events and their significance quite differently to the order in which they actually happened and this is significant. In clinical research we need to know just how people are ordering events and making transformations in time before we can assist them to weave together a story that perhaps, for example, allows them to see events in a more positive, less self-deprecatory way.

If we assume narrative is a powerful cultural discourse, we can examine what a focus on narrative adds to a discourse analysis of people's talk both within and across an interview. We can use narrative analysis to address the generic and individual specificities of speech and to contribute to theory development. Connections with discourse analysis can be made in terms of how participants frame their lives or tell their stories with reference to common, culturally shared ideas about what changes and key events are expected to be made in life. Shared stories can have literary or religious connections, for example, the prodigal son, learning through adversity or a heroic life. In addition, narrative can be investigated from a conversation analytic method, for example, in understanding the situatedness of story production or stories-in-the-telling. Labov and Fanshel's (1977) model of personal experience narratives has found popularity amongst psycho-therapy process researchers, possibly because it approximates the thera-peutic use of personal narrative in therapy. Labov and Fanshel delineate six elements within a narrative: abstract, orientation, action, evaluation, result and coda.

*Steps in the analysis*

1 Read through the transcript a number of times to gain a sense of the person's story. This initial reading can be guided by a drama-based metaphor of people's lives and stories.

2 Note the key features – who are the main protagonists (the main people in the story)? What are the key events or scenes/actions? What is the plot of the story?

3 Make a note of what the dominant theme/story appears to be, perhaps starting to make connections with wider culturally shared stories – the prodigal son, triumph over adversity, and so on.

4 Reflectively note how you may be making connections with your own experiences, how you have become aware of feelings and images as you read the story. How evocative is their story? What aspects evoke particular feelings in you?

5 How is the person telling their story? People express feelings, may become animated, sad, happy, laugh and so on, as they tell their story.

6 Note the variety of stories and themes that emerge from the narratives that people tell. There may be a dominant theme or story that changes at different points in a person's life, for example, a time when things were going well.

7 Significant events or turning points. We can look for events that seemed to mark a change in a person's life or are seen as significant in forming the person that they have become.

8 Coherence. We can focus on many aspects of the narrative in terms of its form and style. One point of focus can be on whether the events as told fit together or appear coherent. This can have a number of components:

- Temporal – whether the events described make sense over time or are scattered and contradictory.
- Semantic – whether the events make sense or whether there are clear contradictions in how events or people are described.

Overall it is important to look for examples where there is a fit between how events are labelled semantically and the episodes that are offered to illustrate them. For example, in telling their story a person may describe a parent as kind but offer very few examples of kindness on their part, or even in contrast, examples of where they have been quite unkind or cruel. This may suggest that they are attempting to edit their own story in ways that are more emotionally bearable for them.

9 Language and discourse. Frequently people's ability to be coherent and clear in their use of language may change at points where very significant events have occurred. Here narrative analysis overlaps with discourse analysis in exploring how feelings are revealed in the way we use language when we describe our lives. For example, the frequency of hesitations may increase, sentences may not be completed, people may hop from one topic to the next without completing them or there may be inappropriate laughter or nervous coughing, perhaps indicating that the person is talking about difficult events. (These are also important clues to the ethics of an interview – see Chapter 9.)

Not all narrative research formally contains all of these components in the analysis but, as we can see, they do offer an analysis which can combine features of discursive and theme analyses into a broader picture of the person and their life. Such a contextualized account gives a view of the person and their life, and is a feature of clinical work and, arguably, of case study research and case reports (see Chapter 7).

*Design*: Either groups or individuals might be interviewed. The interviews usually start in an open-ended manner, inviting participants to tell their stories. However, there may be use of prompts to direct attention to certain areas of interest, such as changes and key events in their lives. For example, high and low points, particularly significant or life-changing events and changes in their sense of self.

*Results*: These are typically presented in terms of the content of people's narratives, along with commonalities about how people make sense of changes. There will also be an analysis of differences in the forms of narratives that people employ. There is likely to be an emphasis on connecting narratives with specific events in people's lives and some generalizations about how events, such as the end of a relationship, can alter these narratives about ourselves.

## QUALITATIVE OBSERVATION

There are a number of reasons for choosing qualitative observation:

- The researcher is interested in meaning in social behaviour as expressed through verbal and non-verbal interactions.
- The researcher relies on observation as an interpretative activity rather than a structured approach to coding frequencies or duration of defined behaviours.
- The researcher wants to generate process observations that describe and explain sequences of social behaviour and contribute to theory development.

An example of qualitative observation is outlined in Research Example 4.8

**Research Example 4.8**

Vetere, A. and Gale, A. (1987) *Ecological Studies of Family Life*. Chichester: Wiley.

This in-depth study explored the nature of interactions in families who had presented with child-focused problems. A participant observation approach was adopted, whereby a researcher lived with a family on two separate occasions, one week at a time. During this time she engaged in the full range of family activities, such as meal times and outings, and domestic duties and leisure activities, such as watching television and playing games. The researcher kept detailed notes of the family members' interactions and, using a structural systemic format, noted the family structure: family boundaries, subsystems, hierarchy, alliances and 'taking sides'. In addition, detailed notes were kept of the experience of the family: the emotional atmosphere, impact on the researcher and inferences about the possible experiences of the family members.

The study suggested that family dynamics as observed in homes were analogous to those typically observed in family therapeutic sessions. However, the timing and pacing were on a different time scale. For example, arguments, disagreements, sulking and so on could last for days rather than the accelerated pace of events in therapy. The analysis of family beliefs was attempted with a repertory grid analysis, which confirmed that the family dynamics were significantly shaped by the nature of the families' beliefs. These had stability and were, for example, the basis of patterns of scapegoating that could occur in the family. A wide range of gender stereotyped behaviours and ideas also became evident as part of the observations, such as implicit expectations about domestic roles, duties and obligations.

## Description of the method

Qualitative observation does not rely predominantly on verbal data but rather on observations of people's actions, decisions, relationships and so on. It is assumed that meanings are expressed and communicated not just by the content of talk but also by behaviours, episodes and rituals, including the detailed analysis of non-verbal behaviours, gestures, posture, expressions and movement. It can also include an analysis of ways of talking, such as tone of voice, pitch, loudness and para-linguistic features (sighs, grunts, coughs and so on). Qualitative observation assumes that we engage in an interpretative process in forming understandings about these features and, like the analysis of language, that we need both to utilize and reflect on them. We write in more detail about these methods in Chapter 8.

*Method*: This may be of individuals or groups of people. Frequently the studies are concerned with observing behaviours in groups such as families, couples or work groups. For example, studies have been conducted to explore how non-verbal communication in couples can lead to escalation or resolution of conflicts.

*Results*: These are usually presented in terms of descriptions of characteristic patterns of interactions. They may include a combination of verbatim sequences of conversation with accompanying description and analysis of non-verbal behaviours. There may also be pictorial representation of non-verbal behaviours and sequences of interaction.

# CASE STUDY

There are a number of reasons for choosing a case study:

- It provides a holistic picture which can allow clinical complexity
- It uses multiple sources of materials
- It is possible to incorporate it as part of clinical work with clients
- It enables the researcher to explore the process of clinical change and intervention
- It provides the opportunity to explore causal factors in the process of change.

An example of a case study is given in Research Example 4.9.

---

**Research Example 4.9**

Stiles, W.B., Meshot, C.M., Anderson, T.T. and Sloan, W.W. (1992) Assimilation of problematic experiences: the case of John Jones, *Psychotherapy Research*, 2(2), 81–101.

The assimilation model proposes a systematic sequence of changes in the representation of a problematic experience during psychotherapy. The authors examined the process of assimilation, tracing changes across 20 sessions in the published transcripts of the psychotherapy of a 25-year-old man. After preparing a catalogue of topics discussed in this treatment, three insights that the client was judged to have were identified in sessions 6, 10 and 14. Using the topic catalogue, the authors searched backwards and forward through the transcripts and selected passages for topics related to the three insights. These passages were assessed qualitatively for the degree of assimilation exhibited. By assessing change in specific ideas, this new approach circumvents conceptual and methodological problems of assessing clients' global long-term change.

---

*Descriptions of the method*

The case study method attempts to consider participants in terms of the complexities of their social and cultural contexts, relationships, work, life events, age, gender and so on. It is an attempt to produce an in-depth, holistic picture of participants in order to make sense of their situations. Case studies also emphasize that knowledge about participants results from an interaction and development of a relationship between researcher and participants. The material for a case study can include verbal data, field observation, case files and reports.

*Design*: This usually involves a study of a case or a series of cases that characterize a particular topic. The cases are chosen to represent particular areas of interest, for example, the experience of becoming a refugee. Typically, several interviews and observations are conducted over a period of time.

*Results*: These are usually detailed descriptions of individuals using qualitative, quantitative or mixed methods approaches. The complexity of each person's experience is featured but generalizations may be drawn, for example, by choosing participants who embody some particularly important or unusual features. For example, forensic studies have been conducted on people who have committed multiple murders or have survived disaster situations.

## THE PROS AND CONS OF THE DIFFERENT QUALITATIVE METHODS

In summary, the different qualitative approaches to data collection and data analysis are not always distinct and may be employed in combinations, as long as the rationale is clear and supports the research question. For example, an observational analysis may complement an interview study, a case study might contain both narrative and observational data, while an interview study might subject the data to both a grounded and a discursive analysis.

Case study and narrative research are more likely to be able to deliver some ideas about causal events and capture the complexity of clinical phenomena. However, they are likely to require more time and commitment from participants.

Thematic analyses (e.g. IPA) offer a picture of the dominant beliefs and schemas of groups and do not demand too much of participants' time. However, they do assume that participants are aware and able to reflect on their experience, which may not be justified in some cases, for example, where participants have experienced events that they are ashamed of or if they are not very verbally able.

Discourse analysis is able to explore subtexts that may underlie how people justify their actions and connect these to wider culturally shared discourses. However, it does not allow us to generalize about enduring beliefs that people may hold. Both IPA and narrative analysis hold a view that people have relatively stable and enduring views about the world and themselves, although arguably narrative approaches are closer to how people talk and think about their lives, in terms of stories, plots, drama and so on.

Observational approaches, especially qualitative studies, have been less in evidence in psychotherapy research, though some forms of discourse analysis, such as rhetorical analysis, include some analysis of non-verbal aspects of speech. It is important to note, however, that clinical work invariably makes use of observational material and that this becomes increasingly central when we move from studying individuals to couples or families. Social psychology and early systemic ideas have emphasized that communication consists of a verbal and non-verbal component and that the congruence between the two is central in helping us to make interpretations. Arguably, observation can be woven in as a component of any of the qualitative methods.

## KEY REFERENCES

Charmaz, K. (1995) Grounded theory, in J. A. Smith, R. Harre and L. van Langenhove (eds) *Rethinking Methods in Psychology*. London: Sage.

Elliot, R., Fischer, C. T. and Rennie, D. L. (1999) Evolving guidelines for publication of qualitative research studies in psychology and related fields, *British Journal of Clinical Psychology*, 38: 215–29.

Glaser, B. G. and Strauss, A. L. (1967) *The Discovery of Grounded Theory: Strategies for Qualitative Research*. Chicago: Aldine.

Hollway, W. (1989) *Subjectivity and Method in Psychology*: *Gender, Meaning and Science*. London: Sage.

Osborn, M. and Smith, J. A. (1998) The personal experience of chronic benign lower back pain: an interpretative phenomenological analysis, *British Journal of Health Psychology*, 3: 65–83.

Vetere, A. and Gale, A. (1987) *Ecological Studies of Family Life*. Chichester: Wiley.

5 ▪ # QUESTIONS OF EVALUATION AND

# OUTCOME

## CHAPTER OVERVIEW

This chapter has been written to encourage clinical practitioners and trainees to take part in more systematic evaluation of their therapeutic work. We are aware that few practitioners engage in formal outcome research and yet, paradoxically almost, they regularly review their work, with their clients, with colleagues in supervision and with themselves (Casement, 1985), using a range of clinical evaluation skills that readily transfer to the research domain. By arguing that our routine clinical review practices constitute the basis of research enquiry, we wish to dismantle the research/practitioner divide, which may have been reinforced by our difficulties in getting started in research and by our beliefs that randomized control trials were the only acceptable form of evaluation research. For most of us, participation in RCTs will not be possible, but participation in small-scale enquiry that extends audit and working in small clinical/research teams that involve service users, in culturally attuned ways, marks the way forward.

This chapter will not outline in detail how to develop measurement tools for small-scale enquiry, such as surveys and questionnaires, as that has been done in Chapters 4, 6, 8 and 9 of this book and with excellence elsewhere (see Robson, 2002). Rather the chapter explores the practical, ethical and theoretical questions and concerns for practitioners and trainees who wish to engage with small-scale research enquiry of an evaluative nature. In particular, we recognize how ongoing evaluation cannot be divorced from an exploration of psychotherapy process. The emphasis here is on do-able research that maximizes participation from all points of view and emphasizes the clinical research skills of practitioners. The chapter includes examples of do-able outcome research in UK NHS working contexts.

## INTRODUCTION

Drawing on Freud's famous technique of word association, we might ask you for a response to the words 'research and psychotherapy'. It is very likely that the responses will be evaluation, outcome and effectiveness. This is perhaps not surprising since we all want to know whether psychotherapy and counselling 'works'. And yet, in our experience, very few psychotherapy practitioners engage in formal evaluation research projects. So, at this point, we should note that Sandberg *et al.* (2002) asked clinical practitioners to identify barriers to their involvement in outcome research. Typical reasons offered included: lack of time and resources; other demands on their time; isolation and lack of peer support; clients' concerns about research participation; a lack of understanding of research methodologies; and, finally, a belief that outcome research is dry and boring! Whilst these findings may not be surprising, they are worrying.

In this chapter we want to review some of the major approaches to evaluation and outcome research, but we also want to focus on ways of conducting such research that are 'do-able'. By this we mean both practically in terms of resources – time, cost and effort – and motivationally in terms of it being of enough interest to want to do it! If, on the other hand, we leave the outcome research to the large-scale randomized control trial (RCT) studies, we shall lose the opportunity to address what the RCTs cannot address, namely understanding what is lost when you pool data and overextend assumptions of generalizability.

## DOES PSYCHOTHERAPY WORK?

### The randomized control trials of psychotherapy outcome

One of the major methods of evaluation of outcome and effectiveness has been the randomized control trials (RCTs) – sometimes referred to as the 'gold standard' of outcome research. The central feature of such research is that participants are randomly assigned to the different conditions in which the researchers are interested. In effect, RCTs attempt to follow the principles of experimental science as developed by Fisher (1935) in relation to research in agriculture. He developed multivariate research designs that examined how different fertilizers, soil types or varieties of grain affected crop yields. By analogy, fertilizers represent therapies, grain represents people and crop yields represent the therapeutic gains! Research Example 5.1 illustrates the use of a RCT design in the evaluation of psychotherapy outcome.

---

**Research Example 5.1**

Leff *et al*. (2000) The London Depression Intervention Trial. Randomised control trial of antidepressants vs couple therapy in the treatment and maintenance of people with depression living with a critical partner: clinical outcome and costs, *British Journal of Psychiatry*, 177: 95–100.

This study compared three approaches for the treatment of severe depression: CBT (cognitive behaviour therapy), systemic couples therapy and drug treatment. Participants volunteered to take part in the study on the basis that they would be randomly allocated to any one of the three approaches. The clinicians delivering each of the approaches were not involved in the process of allocation. This was an attempt to reduce any potential biases in allocating participants that could influence the results. The treatments were manualized so that it was clear what each approach consisted of and also that the different clinicians delivering each approach were consistent and comparable in what they did with each client. Attempts were also made to ensure compatibility between the treatments by controlling for a range of variables, such as the total time spent in treatment. The participants were couples where one partner had been identified as suffering with severe and chronic depression as measured by the BDI (Beck Depression Inventory) and other indicators. It was made clear that they would be randomly allocated to one of three conditions: systemic couples therapy, a programme of CBT or drug therapy with some support and information. Attempts were made to ensure that the amounts of personal contact were similar in the three conditions.

One of the findings of this study was that there was such a high rate of attrition (drop-out) from the CBT part of the study that comparisons were not possible. However, the systemic couples therapy was found to produce more favourable outcomes on a range of measures, including the BDI, than the control group (drug treatment). Interestingly it was also found that independent observers who did not know which partner of each couple had the diagnosis of depression could not reliably identify who had been initially diagnosed. In addition to the outcome findings, this pointed to the validity of a systemic analysis of depression as residing not simply within one partner but as a feature of their relationship.

The 'control' part of the phrase RCT refers not only to the attempts to control a range of potential variables but also to a group which receives no active treatment. This is typically ethically inappropriate in therapy and counselling studies since people experiencing high levels of distress require support and intervention and should not be denied this simply for purposes of the research. One solution is to employ naturally occurring situations, such as clients on waiting lists, who are compared to those who are receiving treatment. In the London Depression Intervention Trial outlined above, in effect the control group were those who were receiving treatment 'as usual', that is medication with some emotional support.

The randomized control trials of therapy treatment outcome have established the evidence base for the major models of psychotherapy (Bergin, 2003). A shorthand summary of the RCT findings has been termed the 'Dodo' verdict'. Broadly, most forms of psychotherapy work and produce better results than no treatment and also produce better results than placebo treatment, which in turn produce better results than no treatment. A placebo treatment is where a condition is devised that superficially looks like a treatment but in fact attempts not to contain the 'active' ingredients of therapy. For example, it has been found in drug trials that being given a placebo drug, such as a sugar pill, could produce change because people expected that it would make them better. Likewise, with psychotherapy and counselling research, the placebo condition is designed to explore the effect of positive expectations on outcome. The approach to outcome studies has been to gain an overall picture by looking at how many studies indicate whether, and how much, psychotherapy is effective.

## Meta-analysis of RCT research

Another approach, called meta-analysis, is to combine the data from a range of studies and subject it to a new analysis, as if the data all came from one big outcome study. In order to do this, the studies have to be comparable in terms of participants, types of problems and measures of change. Such meta-analyses of various RCT outcome studies have directed our attention to the process of psychotherapy (see Chapter 6). It would seem from the meta-analytic studies that the therapeutic relationship and client and therapist resources account for more of the variance in outcome than the specific model of psychotherapy employed (Strupp, 1986). In response to this, RCT study designs have evolved to answer questions of what model of psychotherapy helps certain people, with certain problems, living in certain circumstances (Roth and Fonagy, 1996).

Despite this evolution, some clinicians are still sceptical around the RCT outcome evidence, arguing that for the most part it does not help them make decisions in the specific instance of working with one client; nor does the evidence show that everyone benefits satisfactorily (Lask and Vetere, 2003). So psychotherapy works, for the most part, but it does not seem to help everyone all the time. Most RCT studies of psychotherapy outcome claim benefit for about two-thirds to three-quarters of therapy trial participants and often cannot explore the so-called 'statistical outliers' within the study measures, that is, those people who appear to do very well, or very badly, in terms of the outcome measures. In fact, the statistical outliers may even be excluded from the analysis because they skew the data. As clinicians we want to know what happens to those people who are not helped by our therapy approaches. We would argue that small-scale qualitative studies are helpful in exploring and understanding their experiences (see Chapter 4). There is still a place for clinical judgement, and small-scale investigations, in fitting the research evidence with the theory, alongside what people want and what they say helps them.

Our experience of working within the UK NHS leads us to believe that we, with many of our colleagues, often practise within integrative and conceptually eclectic approaches, whereas by and large the major RCT studies have focused on demonstrating the efficacy of one of the major models of psychotherapy. We are not convinced that all clinicians adhere with loyalty to only one of the major models of psychotherapy. Although we have been identified in our careers with the systemic psychotherapies, as clinical psychologists we are trained in other models of psychotherapy, such as the cognitive therapies, behaviour therapies and brief focal psychodynamic psychotherapies. Thus we wish to encourage practitioners to explore their mix of experiential, theoretical and empirical learning, drawing on the strengths of the evidence base. In this way, and in this chapter, we wish to be seen as even-handed in our approach to the evaluation of the evidence for the major models of counselling and psychotherapy.

## Effectiveness and do-able evaluation research

We shall not outline here the criteria for a good RCT study of therapy outcome, as that has been done very well elsewhere (Barker *et al.*, 2002). Rather we shall turn our attention to the issue of effectiveness and do-able evaluation research. We find our approach to therapy practice is increasingly integrative in practice, anchored in formulation that is at the very least contextualized! And this evolution in ourselves, mirrors the concern we have about the major RCT studies, namely that they are usually model specific. We agree that we need to be accountable for our psychotherapy practice, to all our stakeholders, both in our theory base and our evidence base. But many of the RCT studies (on which we rely for our evidence base) have been conducted with the backing of large research grants and the resources that large grants can buy, which is out of the reach of most of us. Additionally, RCT studies tend to work in highly structured therapy trials contexts, with research therapists and with populations of people who do not always resemble the groups who seek therapy in our working contexts.

They speak to efficacy rather than effectiveness. Their internal validity is always high, but external validity is often questionable (see Research Example 5.1 as a noted exception).

Most of us cannot rigorously select clients for participation in outcome research, nor can we recruit enough participants to meet the requirements of power analysis for statistical comparisons. We often wish to focus on the impact of change beyond symptom reduction, and the client's activity is crucial to what we can and cannot do, for example, with missed sessions, completing self-report diaries and so on. Thus this chapter develops some ideas about how we can build a practice base of evidence that may be local to us, utilizing our available resources, such as participating with colleagues and service users in small clinical/research teams, and speaking to the needs of our client groups and our purchasers. In addition, the major RCT studies have established a retrospective evidence base, in that they have evaluated established approaches to psychotherapy and counselling practice. As practitioners we may want to evaluate our own adaptations of existing models or our creative leaps of practice. Individual case study approaches may be ideally suited to this task (see Chapter 7). Case studies can provide powerful descriptions of what seems to be important for people in the process of change. These descriptions can inform subsequent experiential and empirical enquiry. Repeated case studies offer an opportunity to test hypotheses about what works and what does not work in relation to therapeutic outcomes: both the accumulation of evidence and disconfirmation! The studies and methods we feature in this chapter have application for practitioners in the NHS and private practice, with limited resources and limited time, and for practitioners undertaking Masters and Doctoral training programmes that have a research component.

## EVIDENCE: EVIDENCE BASED PRACTICE AND PRACTICE BASED EVIDENCE

We have written elsewhere in detail of our particular weave of formulation, intervention and evaluation in our therapeutic work (Vetere and Dallos, 2003). At the heart of our approach is the notion that formulation is the vehicle for integrative practice and the friend of evaluation. Formulation is an ongoing process, of seeking and processing feedback from our clients and our clinical experiences, such that thinking is informed in a recursive loop with practice. This is the basis on which we can hold ourselves accountable and explore the nature of therapeutic understanding and change. It is also the basis on which we can be seen to engage in the constant evaluation of our work. You cannot formulate unless you evaluate!

Psychotherapy has received many challenges as to its viability and legitimacy. One response has been to produce data to support the case that it works. As we say above, the most widely promoted case has been made in terms of RCT studies. However, this begs many questions about what constitutes *evidence*. In the following chapters we will see many varieties of evidence for different kinds of studies. Broadly we can divide these into studies that produce qualitative data and those that produce quantitative data (see Table 5.1). As we have seen in Chapter 2, in formulating our research questions we need to consider questions about what we want to know. This connects with what kind of data we wish to gather. Simply put, this boils down to whether we are seeking to have data that allow quantifications and some use of numbers and statistics or data that are more concerned with meanings and descriptions. In effect, a piece of research and an evaluation are as good as the data we have available – what we have chosen to measure (see our discussion in Chapter 1 of the meaning of mental health).

**Table 5.1**    Characteristics of quantitative and qualitative data

| Quantitative | Qualitative |
| --- | --- |
| Numbers, statistics | Meanings, themes |
| Objective data | Subjective data |
| Nomothetic | Idiographic |
| Measurable | Interpretative |
| Expert | Collaborative |

We are not intent on encouraging a separation between these two types of data, but it helps to find a starting point for thinking about what we seek to gain from an evaluation or outcome study. Typically, such studies have been associated with quantitative data, on the premise that an assessment of how effective an approach is requires data in the form of quantification and numbers. Critical to the question of what types of data we collect is our understanding of the process of change in psychotherapy and counselling. The question in effect is: in what ways can we capture that change has occurred, and to what extent can we measure this?

Pinsof and Wynne (2000) argue that every therapy process moment can also be seen as an outcome. If we can identify moments during the actual therapy, or in reflecting on ourselves outside the therapy room, where we act, think and feel differently – 'the differences that make a difference' (Bateson, 1972, p. 110) – we can be said to be aware of our process of change. Such a view helps us think beyond therapy outcomes as discrete measurable events, fixed in time, to thinking of them as fluid, dialectical and subject to change in their own right. This is a revolutionary view. It opens the way to accept experiential, theoretical and empirical evidence for our therapeutic practice as having equal legitimacy, in that it suggests that clinicians can from their own experience, from talking to service users, as much as they can from externally imposed ideas and others' findings. This has implications for what we might choose to measure when thinking of outcomes: symptom change; subjective well-being; the subjective feelings of others; others' observations of themselves and of us; and collective measures, such as repertory grids.

## First order and second order change

Those readers familiar with the systemic psychotherapy literature will need no introduction to the terms first order and second order change. However, for readers whose practice orientation does not include these terms, we have included them here as they are crucial to how we might approach the issue of evaluating our therapies.

First order change refers to those changes believed to be made as a result of engagement in therapy, such as behavioural changes, changes in our attitudes and beliefs and so on. These changes are often referred to in the outcome literature as 'symptom reduction' and may be measured pre-, during or post-therapy, using simple questionnaires, such as the BECK II, the HADS, the GHQ-12, and so on. (See Chapter 9 for a description of how to design brief outcome/satisfaction questionnaires, or Robson, 2002, for a fuller description.)

Second order change, on the other hand, refers to the wider relational effects of the therapy, for the client, their colleagues, carers and significant others, and for their relationships. Clearly these wider impacts, such as relational effects, are harder to capture and measure. But for those of us who work with individuals living in significant relationships, we are keen to know how individual change impacts on their relationship well-being. We may be working with couples; we may be working with individuals and invite partners to participate in partner-assisted treatment approaches; we may be working with parents/carers and children; we may be consulting to a staff team and want to explore changes in team functioning alongside any felt improvement in well-being or reduction in stress. So, when we want to explore the wider impacts of our therapeutic work, we need to find ways to move beyond pre- and post-intervention individual symptom measures to give some indication of group changes in functioning. This is where single case study exploration through multiple interviews, and pilot explorations using different data sources, can be most helpful to the development of clinical research hypotheses. The current climate in the social sciences is pluralist, with respect to the theory and method of research practice. Psychotherapy and counselling researchers have led the way in adapting and fitting the methods of research to the clinical phenomena they wish to study. There is recognition that one methodological size does not fit all.

Our first task as psychotherapy and counselling researchers is to identify how individuals and groups learn and maintain therapeutic changes outside the therapy sessions. To do this, we look to the social science disciplines of psychology, sociology and anthropology for their theories of individual and social group learning, often rooted in both observation and laboratory based studies. In bringing together our clinical wisdom with the social science research, we look at the fit: to what extent does our understanding of the nature and process of therapy change fit with what our social science colleagues have discovered? This has implications for the kinds of data we collect, the crucial role of pilot enquiry, and for seeing method as the servant of enquiry. We would recommend that, where possible, we fit observational measures alongside self-report measures, thus capturing multiple perspectives and triangulating our findings with different types of data (see Chapters 8 and 10).

## THEORY AND THE PROBLEM OF THE FOLLOW-UP PERIOD

When AV was teaching a module on 'Researching the Family' to psychology Research Methods Masters students, she did a session on researching the outcomes of family therapy, which included the RCT studies. During the session, the students were invited to critique the RCT rationales and methodologies as part of their teaching and learning. One of the issues that always troubled AV was the matter of the follow-up to the therapy and the period of time used to conduct the follow-up. Whilst believing follow-up was important for showing the 'enduring' nature of therapeutic change, AV was never convinced of the theoretical window assumed within the follow-up period. So, if a study used a typical nine-month, or one-year follow-up period, could changes reported at the end of therapy still evident later on perhaps be attributed to the therapy process? If a study used an 18- or 24-month follow-up period in the expectation of continuing to track therapeutic changes, and they were not still found, rather than assuming the therapy had limited impact, should we ask to what extent theoretically speaking, a therapy could or should be expected to show continuing changes? What is the model of change the therapy theory uses that would predict continuing change at 18 months post-therapy, say? Instead, we might argue that 'life' takes over where the therapy leaves off, and a person gets more involved in positively reinforcing events within their own social worlds, facilitated by their therapy experiences. Such a view lends itself to the notion of social and psychological change as a fundamental and fluid process, punctuated by a therapy moment, which joins the interplay of forces, both internal and external that help in shaping our social realities. Thus any attempt we make to understand the nature and process of change in our psychotherapeutic work contributes to our knowledge about outcomes.

### Collaborative practice

This chapter aims to show how in many ways we cannot separate questions of process from outcome. This leads on to collaborative practice, for if we see process moments as mini-outcomes, we need to understand all participants' points of view in order to begin untangling what might be going on. And therein lies the rub. Conducting research enquiry that seeks multiple perspectives, with perhaps multiple sources of data, stretches our existing methodologies. It offers opportunities for counselling and psychotherapy researchers to adapt their tried and tested clinical methods of enquiry to the more formal exigencies of the research enquiry, for example, theory-practice linking; assessment questions that link multiple views; therapeutic questioning practices that can be adapted for research interviews; formulation practices; therapy reviews; observation; interpretative activity; and so on.

Research Example 5.2 illustrates an innovative and collaborative approach to data collection in the service of promoting understanding with small-scale outcomes.

**Research Example 5.2**

Vostanis, P., Burnham, J. and Harris, Q. (1992) Changes of expressed emotion in systemic family therapy, *Journal of Family Therapy*, 14(1): 15–27.

This study explored changes in expressed emotion (EE; Leff and Vaughn, 1985) as a result of family involvement in systemic family therapy. Video-tapes of the therapy were rated for the first, second and final sessions, for 12 families, by an independent rater, trained in the rating of expressed emotion, so defined. Six of the therapies had been completed before the study began and six were rated prospectively. Emotional overinvolvement and criticism were found to decrease significantly from the early stages of the work, whilst warmth was found to increase later.

   This is an interesting example of a do-able study, within the time scale of a doctoral research project that adapts an established rating scheme (EE) to another context, and which has been shown to have ability in other therapy contexts to predict whether individuals and families complete treatment and otherwise derive benefits.

## ETHICS AND ACCOUNTABILITY: RCTS AND THE PROBLEM OF THE 'ETHICAL' CONTROL GROUP

As psychotherapy providers, we do need to be accountable for our practice. Most of us root our accountability within our use of theory and draw on the extant evidence base (usually RCT based, but not always) to justify our services. Clinical governance procedures adopted throughout the UK NHS require us to show how we use the existing evidence base to inform our practice and to show that we are delivering the best possible service. But, we also need to engage with the common complaints that RCT study findings lag behind advances in clinical innovation and cannot tell us *what* is going on in the therapy, what people are doing in therapy and how to promote the outcomes we all seek.

   Here we would like to consider group comparison outcome research that does not use a control group and is managed on a low budget. It has been argued elsewhere (Sloane *et al.*, 1975) that high levels of ethical concern can be maintained with careful monitoring of people in the control group and provision of treatment on demand if they are found to be distressed. However, we now find ourselves in a position of having an evidence base for the major models of psychotherapy and so no longer need the ethical wait list control group, so called. Newer variants of therapy that still need to show their effectiveness can proceed with an accumulation of evidence using small-scale case study designs, both quantitative and qualitative. When sufficient case study evidence accumulates, those treatments can be compared with the more established treatments, as happened with the recent London Depression Intervention Trial, where individuals with a diagnosis of severe depression were allocated to one of three conditions:

pharmacotherapy, cognitive behaviour therapy or systemic couples therapy (Leff *et al.*, 2000; see Research Example 5.1).

Bennun's research, published in 1986, provides us with a good example of do-able group comparison design outcome research conducted within the time scale of a PhD study (see Research Example 5.3).

---

### Research Example 5.3

Bennun, I. (1986) Evaluating family therapy: a comparison of the Milan and problem-solving approaches, *Journal of Family Therapy*, 8: 225–42 .

Bennun mounted a comparative study of the effectiveness of one model of family therapy with another – Milan family therapy and problem solving family therapy. Twenty families were assigned over a three-year period to either of the treatment conditions, for a maximum of ten sessions. Initially he had intended to study families with a member with a drinking problem, but recruitment problems meant that he needed to include other presenting problems, such as depression, eating problems and some child focused problems.

The study measured outcomes at three levels:

1 symptomatic change pre- and post-therapy using a variety of standardized measures, such as the Beck Depression Inventory (Beck, 1967) and the Severity of Alcohol Dependence Questionnaire (Stockwell *et al.*, 1983);
2 family system change was assessed with a modified version of the Shapiro Personal Questionnaire (Shapiro, 1975);
3 family members rated their satisfaction with treatment on a five-point scale, along with whether their initial concerns had remained the same, increased or decreased.

The measures employed tried to separate outcome and satisfaction; to measure both symptom and system change (see above for a description of first and second order change); and to incorporate family members' views of outcome. Measures were taken pre-therapy, during the therapy, post-therapy and at six-month follow-up.

The results indicated that both groups appeared to benefit overall, in that they all reported symptom reduction, although the Milan group seemed to show more evidence of systemic change.

Criticisms of the study include: the use of a small sample; a lack of process monitoring for the therapists; one therapist for the Milan family therapy and five therapists for the problem solving approach; families were not randomly assigned to the two therapy groups; the assessment of systemic change were not carried out 'blind' to the treatment group the family were in. This study, whilst suffering from some problems with internal validity, was high in external validity, in that it involved working with 'real' NHS clients, 'real' NHS therapists and in 'real' NHS settings. It can be commended for its use of a follow-up telephone questionnaire that asked for information both about satisfaction and outcome progress.

## COMPLETING THE AUDIT CYCLE

In our experience, most of us groan when we hear the word 'audit'. We are never sure quite why, unless it is in anticipation of some meaningless counting activity, imposed on us by others, that does not help us as clinicians (Maclachlan and Newnes, 2002). But, we all do audit! Many psychotherapy and counselling practitioners will routinely ask clients questions before, during and at the end of sessions – questions that monitor the nature of change, the well-being of the therapeutic alliance and the progress of sessions (Barnard and Kuehl, 1995). For example, we might ask for 'updates', what was helpful or unhelpful about the last session, or this session, and what else needs to happen. Since we ask these questions in a regular and ongoing way, we and our clients are uniquely positioned to adjust and alter the flow and nature of the sessions as we follow the feedback. The questions and the responses can be recorded in the clinical notes after our sessions, or during our sessions if we work collaboratively with our clients to record progress, change and stuckness. Our sessions may be audio-taped or video-taped, and if we work in clinical teams, the evaluation conversation may be noted during the session. Such conversations invite our clients to articulate and develop their own ideas about progress and change in relation to our developing ideas. The conversations and notes can be content analysed or searched for themes that help hone research questions and develop clinical research hypotheses (see Chapters 2 and 4). The difference between audit and routine clinical practice, therefore, may simply lie in how systematically we enquire about these matters, how the information is held and recorded and who else gets to know.

In the UK, the Clinical Governance agenda has continued to develop. Audit measures of outcome have been developed that satisfy the needs of management, such as costs of a service, waiting list management and 'throughput' in a service. Many clinicians find such measures to be poor indicators of the quality of the care offered and the quality of the clinical outcomes. The Health of the Nation Scales (Wing *et al.*, 1998) were developed in part to try to find a way of objectively measuring the clinical impact of our work with clients. Burbidge *et al.* (2004) would say that these measures do not go far enough. They give as an example the work of Cheseldine (1995), who developed the Goal Attainment Scale as a way of trying to quantify clinical objectives, monitor clinical progress and analyse the quality of clinical care. It has the sensitivity clinicians look for to help them monitor care and enable their further professional development, but it has the disadvantage of not being helpful to purchasers. The data produced are not easily used for purposes of comparison.

Burbidge *et al.* (2004) responded to these dilemmas by developing an outcome measure that both satisfied the organization's need for audit by producing quantitative data, and providing data that would help clinicians positively shape their own work. They developed a data recording sheet that identified the client's diagnosis (using ICD-10) and presenting problems, in the following categories: cognitions, sensory, emotional, behavioural, daily living skills and social skills. For each presenting problem, the clinician made a series of ratings using five-point Likert scales:

- case ratings – provided information about chronicity and complexity of the presenting problem(s) and compliance with the intervention;
- need ratings – provided information about frequency, intensity and unpredictability of the presenting problem/s; and
- impact ratings – provided information about the presenting problem(s) on the quality of life of clients and their significant relationships.

They developed written guidelines for completing the measures on the data recording sheet. The guidelines lend themselves to independent assessment of the reliability of the use of the data recording sheet. For example, two clinicians can assess the same person, couple or family. The data recording sheet can be filled in prior to treatment, during treatment and at the end of treatment to give a flavour of progress – or lack of progress.

The above example lends itself to auditing our work with individual clients in adult mental health settings. The work of Reimers and Treacher (1995) is an example of regular audit with family groups who attended child and adolescent mental health services (CAMHS). As two practising clinicians, they did not have the time (nor the funds to employ a research assistant) to conduct a regular and thorough audit. They were able to use the help of a psychology student, placed with them in the third year of her studies, on a work placement, as part of a four-year undergraduate degree. The student interviewed family members, with permission, in their own homes following the end of the family work. As an independent interviewer she was able to ask them about their experiences of the family work, what they found helpful and unhelpful, and so on. These interviews were conducted in three waves, with each wave producing findings that the clinicians were able to implement at work, thus completing the audit cycle. As an example, the first wave of follow-up interviews found that many family members did not like the use of the one-way screen and team (behind the screen), and felt uncomfortable because they did not know who the team members were, nor their intentions. Subsequently, the team decided to make themselves more visible, introducing themselves at the start of the work, and continually being 'present' during the work, with the therapists referring to them by name and so on. The second wave of interviews found a marked improvement in family members' comfort with the use of a screen and team.

Another example from the same set of audit studies can be found in the team's wish to understand why some families did not attend their appointments. Their 'did not attend' rate was about the same as might be expected in a CAMHS: one in three families did not attend their first appointment. The second wave of interviews found that family members were initially frightened that the team would be in a social services department and would be likely to remove the children from their care, showing how sometimes people do not always understand the distinctions between our statutory services. The second fear they held was that they would be blamed for their child's difficulties. This finding led the team to put these concerns 'on the table for discussion' at the start of their meetings. It also encouraged one of the team members, with permission, to seek to visit families at home to introduce himself to them and explain a bit about their service prior to their first appointment. This took about 15 minutes of his time, on his way home. Subsequent audit showed that their DNA rate for the first appointment almost dropped to zero as a result. Of course, this brings another problem, as we all recognize, in that we often use our 'missed' appointment times to catch up with our administration, in busy clinics!

## WHOSE VIEW IS IT ANYWAY?

Many therapists and counsellors hold the belief that some therapeutic phenomena and impacts cannot be accessed well by traditional methods – the complexity is reduced, multiple meanings are stripped away or the phenomenon seems to dissolve – as if these phenomena are only made visible when experienced through an emotionally engaged interaction with a therapist observer. As such, our experience of the therapeutic relationship, and our behaviour within it, is an important part of the success or failure of the therapy, because it influences the meaning of the help that is both offered and experienced. Drawing on these multiple meanings and experiences, we would argue, is important in advancing our specific understandings of what helps and why.

Howard *et al.* (1993) would argue that different types of change occur as therapy progresses and that repeat measures of outcome will not only reveal a phased model of psychotherapy but will also help to predict successful progression into later phases of treatment. Their research into outcomes suggests three phases of psychotherapy: re-moralization – or a hopefulness change; remediation – or symptom change; and rehabilitation – or life change. They asked a large sample of individual psychotherapy participants to complete self-report measures of subjective well-being, symptomatic distress and life functioning before the start of therapy and after sessions 2, 4 and 17. The measures generated dichotomous data, and analysis of 2×2 cross-classification tables suggested that improvement in well-being precedes and is a probabilistic necessary condition for reduction in symptomatic distress. It also suggested that symptomatic improvement precedes and is a probabilistic and necessary condition for improvement in life functioning.

## USER VIEWS: INVOLVING CHILDREN IN EVALUATING OUTCOMES

Children's views as direct service users (notwithstanding problematic issues of consent), and as people who live with adults who might be the service users, are important, but historically their views have been neglected. Many practitioners work in child, adolescent and family services, and even more of us work in adult services with adults who are also parents and carers of children. Mullender *et al.* (2002) argue that traditional deficit models of developmental psychology have led to the marginalization of children as a source of information about their own lives. They think children have been conceptualized as 'growing up into the adult world' as if they are somehow incomplete or not yet competent because of their maturational stage. They suggest that childcare policies and practices could be enriched if children were consulted around the design and delivery of services.

Recently the family therapy literature has acknowledged this neglect of children's views and a number of do-able small-scale qualitative research studies have been published, as illustrated by Research Example 5.4.

---

**Research Example 5.4**

Strickland-Clark, L., Campbell, D. and Dallos, R. (2000) Children's and adolescents' views on family therapy, *Journal of Martial Therapy*, 22(3): 324–41.

This study involved interviewing a small sample of children and adolescents (N = 5), immediately following their family therapy sessions, asking about their experiences of helpful and unhelpful events during the therapy sessions. Using semi-structured interviews and video-tape cued recall of the sessions, children identified their significant moments in the therapy. The interviews were analysed using grounded theory (Glaser and Strauss, 1967) and the significant events were analysed using comprehensive process analysis (see Chapter 9 for a description of the CPA). Some interesting themes emerged from the analyses, such as the importance of being heard and the difficulty of being unheard; the importance of being included in the therapy process; facing up to and coping with challenges in the therapy; how therapy brings back painful family memories and thus why children think other family members may not attend; difficulties in saying what you think and feel and concern about others' reactions; needing support in the sessions; and, last but not least, their pleasure in being asked to take part in the interviews!

---

As another example, Lobatto (2002) interviewed six children some three to six months following the end of their outpatient work with a CAMHS team. The children were interviewed at home, in the presence of a parent or carer. The interviews lasted about half an hour, and followed a semi-structured format in which the children were asked about: their understanding of the reasons for attending for family therapy; expectations of them during the meetings; their experiences of feeling heard and understood by others during the meetings; and their ideas about what was happening during the therapy. The interviews were analysed using a grounded theory approach as modified by Charmaz (1995). Lobatto found the children willing and eager to participate in the research interviews. It was noted that the parent/carer who 'sat in' commented that the children spoke more during the research interview than during the therapy meetings – a phenomenon we have noted elsewhere (see Chapter 9). The children seemed to appreciate multiple choice questions, as open questions appeared to raise anxiety. They reported sometimes feeling unsure about the 'rules' of participation in therapy, and described how they moved in and out of the conversation at times, when they felt embarrassed or criticized, for example.

Such findings have helpful implications for practitioners who work with children and families. Agreeing with parents, carers and children, in a culturally attuned way, the ground rules for children's participation in family work and devising strategies to strengthen children's working alliances with both parents and therapists during the sessions would help children manage their participation.

## CULTURALLY ATTUNED RESEARCH

Turner (2000) draws our attention as researchers to assumptions of cultural homogeneity that may underpin our research questions and research designs. Writing in the USA, he argues that a consensus model of cultural and ethnic fusion has not emerged, leaving disparate groups holding on to their own values, beliefs and practices, often rooted in their culture of origin. Because of the importance to us all, of our dearly held cultural beliefs, he asserts that our research designs and methods should properly clarify and appreciate the role of culture, ethnicity and race in problem occurrence, treatment, outcome and prevention. One clear implication is whether and to what extent we routinely consult with our potential research participants, rather than assuming we might be an appropriate arbiter of specific group concerns. Lack of consultation could have led in the past to selection bias in respondents and the use of non-comparable measures. Given that we all have more or less competence in switching between different codes and norms, do RCT studies that pool findings miss an opportunity to address how those in a minority manage within the dominant majority group, and particularly with therapies developed within and for that majority group?

The comparative lack of success in engaging some minority groups with prevention and treatment programmes might suggest the need to develop more sensitivity in our research designs to the multifaceted problems and protective factors faced by those in a minority, and adapt those designs accordingly. This is an area of enquiry where the in-depth, collaborative case study design can help to highlight the specific concerns of the group in question, such as how minority status is conceptualized and experienced and how it impacts on treatment outcomes (albeit indirectly through the mediation of other socio-economic factors). Within this framework, minority status would be conceptualized as an explanatory variable rather than a descriptive variable, making explicit where and how the majority group findings had served as the 'norm' or 'standard' for comparison. This is particularly important in evaluating the outcomes of preventative interventions because the collaboration of participants is needed over extended periods of time and for the non-occurrence of a problem. Groups that are suspicious of the majority group may well not seek services, if at all, until a crisis occurs.

We advocate client focused, learning based research models that explore our day-to-day lived clinical realities, where both client and practitioner are active and interested in exploring outcomes. For an example, see the action research models developed in education research (Bassey, 1998). Research access to minority communities who may have a history of distrust with the majority group demands that we take time to build relationships of trust, promoting collaborative research designs that have clear benefits for the participants themselves. We may use culture as a map, but we need to be sensitive to group differences and even-handed around differences that may be self-defining. Focus groups can help us to explore and pilot relevant outcome research questions and measures that have ecological validity, so that we use participants' understanding of both the problems at hand and good outcomes. In-depth case studies may precede the use of group based comparative designs.

However, a note of caution may be needed. As much as we might advocate principles of collaboration and democratized research processes, we are mindful of Sixsmith's (2004) research with young men from disadvantaged backgrounds. The young men had been excluded from mainstream services and a volunteer group had helped them refurbish a dilapidated council house as their group home. The researchers wanted to know about the young men's health care needs and how they looked after those needs. They tried hard to include the men in the design of the research, but all their attempts were met with jokes, loud music, or quick exits from the room. With some persistence, they found they could some-times have very brief conversations in corridors with the men on their own, but they could never meet their own standards as researchers for participatory community based research design. The men were willing to have the researchers around as observers and provided 'data' as asked, but clearly seemed to position the researchers as the 'experts'.

## CHAPTER SUMMARY: AREAS OF DATA COLLECTION THAT MAKE A DIFFERENCE TO CLINICAL PRACTICE

What data might make a difference to our treatment outcomes and lend themselves to small-scale enquiry? The following are areas of data collection that we think will make a difference to clinical practice and are feasible:

- Data on procedures for engaging individuals, couples, families, work teams and so on in therapeutic work, across diverse cultural traditions and across the lifespan. (For example, outcome research to date would suggest that successful treatment outcomes are mediated by therapist experience to the extent that it is linked to higher success with engagement.) In-depth case studies of mutually beneficial and collaborative therapy relationships will complement the generalized findings of the RCTs (easily digested findings).
- Data on the clients' models of change. What have we learned from listening to what our clients have to say? What have we learned from our own experiences of grappling with depression, anxiety, relationship dilemmas, trauma recovery and so on? How does this knowledge drive our formulation and evaluation questions? What are our motivations for working with a particular client group? Do we make assumptions about majority group homogeneity?

- Data on procedures for understanding exceptions, stuckness and ambivalence to change. What do we do with our feelings and intuitions about the 'right' and 'wrong' way to proceed at certain moments in therapy, and how are they connected to outcomes? In-depth case studies that examine mutually agreed and beneficial solutions.
- Data on procedures for ending therapy and helping to prevent relapse.

## KEY REFERENCES

Barnard, C. P. and Kuehl, B. P. (1995) On-going evaluation: in-session procedures for enhancing the working alliance and therapy effectiveness, *The American Journal of Family Therapy*, 23(2): 161–72.

Burbidge, C., Chamberlain, P. and Gallsworthy, L. (2004) Making outcomes measures work for psychologists, *Clinical Psychology*, 44: 30–33.

Leff, J., Vearnals, S., Brevin, C. R., Wolff, G., Alexander, B., Asen, K., Dayson, D., Jones, E., Chisholm, D. and Everitt, B. (2000) The London Depression Intervention Trial. Randomised control trial of antidepressants vs couple therapy in the treatment and maintenance of people with depression living with a critical partner: clinical outcome and costs. *British Journal of Psychiatry*, 177: 95–100.

Pinsof, W. M. and Wynne, L. C. (2000) Toward progress research: closing the gap between family therapy practice and research, *Journal of Marital and Family Therapy*, 26(1): 1–8.

Reimers, S. and Treacher, A. (1995) *Introducing User-Friendly Family Therapy*. London: Routledge.

Robson, C. (2002) *Real World Research*, 2nd edn. Oxford: Blackwell.

# 6  PSYCHOTHERAPY PROCESS RESEARCH: EXPLORING WHAT HAPPENS IN PSYCHOTHERAPY

## CHAPTER OVERVIEW

This chapter starts with an exploration of the nature of psychotherapy process research and how it is central to the development of our understanding of how therapy works. It moves on to offer a guide for conducting psycho-therapy process research. The book's themes are explored to consider research that is concerned with the meaning and experience of psycho-therapy, that involves a collaboration between participants in the research process and that is do-able in the limited time that most clinicians possess. We consider the advantages and disadvantages of therapists researching their own practice. The chapter then offers an overview of the main types of psychotherapy process research and illustrates how these are located within different theories of how change occurs in therapy. Detailed examples of the main areas of psychotherapy process research are offered as illustrative guides, along with key references.

## INTRODUCTION: WHAT IS PSYCHOTHERAPY PROCESS RESEARCH?

Psychotherapy process research (PPR) aims to consider fundamental questions about how change is achieved in psychotherapy and counselling, along with the broader question of how people achieve change in their lives. Some psychotherapists point out that this is an immense task:

> As therapists we know, subjectively, that the process of psychotherapy is constituted by a multiplicity of interactions, tentative invitations to change, mutual construction of new and old meanings, exploration of difference, resources, creativities, fears and blocks, feedback from previous communications, and so on into an infinity of complexity for which we have some technical description and some explanation, but much of which still resides outside our capacity to capture it and pin it down.
>
> (Jones, 2003, p. 350)

In this chapter we want to consider how research can be faithful to this complexity but, at the same time, try to capture some of the active ingredients of therapy. As with the rest of the book, we want to explore ways of conducting research that are 'do-able' for us as busy clinicians but that still contribute to and build our understanding of psychotherapy and counselling practice. We also want to consider research that is collaborative and emancipatory, in that it is a shared endeavour between researchers, therapists and clients. Perhaps even more so than with other areas of research, we want to aim for research that allows us insights into both client and therapist experiences and their reflections. As we will discuss, one of the most consistent findings from psychotherapy process research is that the relationship between the client and therapist is critical. To gain an understanding of this relationship we need to take an 'insider' perspective, in which we explore the thoughts and feelings of both therapist and client in constructing their relationship.

Many studies have been conducted to show that a whole range of disorders can be ameliorated through psychotherapy, for example, anxiety disorders, depression, eating disorders, obsessive disorders, conduct dis-orders and even psychosis and personality disorder (Bergin and Garfield,

1994; Bergin, 2003). We have summarized some of this body of research (see Chapter 5) and, as we have seen, the conclusions are that the psychotherapies, taken broadly, are more effective than placebo groups and more effective again than no treatment of people on waiting lists. The comparison with placebo groups is important because it suggests that the effects are due to more than an expectation or faith that one will be helped.

As a general rule we can say that psychotherapies can produce significant change in 75 per cent of people treated. But put another way, one in four do not get much better! Acknowledging this general indication of effectiveness, psychotherapy process research asks the important question: how does psychotherapy work? And, related to this, for whom does it not work, and why? We can point out that psychotherapy is not by any means alone in offering assistance without full understanding of how it produces its effects. The history of psychiatry, for example, shows many examples of fortuitous findings in the development of modern psychotropic drugs. We understand less about how they work than the fact that in some cases they appear to offer at least some relief of difficult symptoms and distress.

## Psychotherapy process research questions

Our initial questions clearly are about the process of psychotherapy, but this may be in a form that is general rather than quite specific. For example, we might be interested broadly in the experience of psychotherapy for a particular group, such as children. Alternatively, we might want to start with a much more focused question, such as what specific events in therapy, such as challenging cognitions, promote change in clients' insight into their problem. The kinds of questions we will generate will in turn be influenced by the kinds of psychotherapy research that have been conducted. We may wish to develop a particular form of research or combine several features in order to attempt an investigation. Box 6.1 offers a summary of some of the major varieties of psychotherapy process research that have been conducted.

---

**Box 6.1　Main areas of psychotherapy process research**

**1　Therapeutic alliance** – this has perhaps been the largest area of research into PPR. Studies have explored the nature of the therapeutic relationship, how this appears to be a common active ingredient across a range of therapies, ruptures or breaks in the alliance, how the alliance shifts during therapy and how the early nature of the alliance predicts outcome. One important area of focus has been that ruptures in the therapeutic relationship and their repair indicate important points in therapy.

*Methods*: Observation, inventories, interviews

**2　Analysis of shifts in meanings** – these studies have adopted a broad approach to explore how shifts in understandings occur during therapy. Some have adopted a broad qualitative 'exploratory approach', while others have employed a structured framework, for example, looking at shifts across a range of dimensions of meanings or constructs or, more specifically, at meanings relating more specifically to the presenting problems.

*Methods*: Interview studies, theme analysis, personal questionnaires, pcp, questionnaires

**3    Significant events** – these studies start from the premise that therapeutic change occurs in discrete bursts, a sense that something falls into place at certain moments. This research in some ways connects with the notion of ruptures and repair in the therapeutic alliance research. Typically, people report some sense of being confronted or challenged by different ways of seeing things which helps to transcend established patterns of thinking and feelings. Clients also typically report strong feelings associated with these change points.

*Methods*: Interviews – assisted with audio or video replay (interpersonal process recall), questionnaires

**4    Systemic/process studies** – this represents a broad band of research that has attempted to look at what therapists actually 'do' in sessions as opposed to what they think they do. Initially this contains descriptions of what kinds of things therapists working in different approaches do. For example, CBT therapists work in a more directive way that those using exploratory psychotherapies using ideas from Rogerian therapy or personal construct theory. Included here are studies which have attempted to look specifically at therapy in terms of conversation, for example, the extent to which therapists direct topics of conversation, listen, interrupt, make interpretations and so on. Such research can reveal differences between the theory and practice of therapy, for example, 'exploratory' and non-directive therapies, as in the famous study of Rogers' work (Truax, 1966).

*Methods*: Observation, analysis of transcripts, interviews

**5    Client and therapist variables** – this includes studies that have attempted to examine differences between therapists, for example, to explore and compare the actions of 'experts', with a proven record of success, as opposed to novice therapists. The intention is to generate ideas that might point to some fundamental features of what constitutes 'good' therapy.

*Methods*: Outcome measures of therapy, inventories to measure client and therapist variables

**6    Interpersonal models of change** – these explore the fit between client and therapist factors. As an example, the impact of the client's and therapist's previous histories can be explored to see how the therapeutic relationship can offer new ways of relating which promote change.

*Methods*: Structured observation, inventories

> **7   Cycle of change** – this is based on the idea that different therapeutic approaches need to be employed since clients vary in their ability to engage in the process of change. These studies connect with the assimilation model but regard change as a cyclical process.

## PROCESS RESEARCH AND THEORIES OF CHANGE

Most therapies are informed by particular theoretical lenses which contain models of the person, including psychological, sociological and ethical aspects. Related to this, various theories have ideas about how problems develop and concomitant ideas about how change is achieved. Our chosen theory directs us to search in some places and not in others. For example, research into cognitive therapies takes as its primary focus changes in behaviours, cognitive schemas and negative automatic thoughts. In contrast, the transpersonal therapies see changes in relation to shifts in autonomy, self-actualization and authenticity. This raises the possibility that any psychotherapy, and possibly process research into these approaches, may bring with it a theoretical position. However, the theories of change that drive the practice of a particular approach may not necessarily correspond with what clients experience as being helpful in enabling them to change. Furthermore, what therapists actually do in practice may differ from what their theory of psychotherapy suggests they should be doing. (See Table 6.1.)

**Table 6.1**   Theories of change

| | | | | |
|---|---|---|---|---|
| *Types of change:* | Cognitive | Behavioural | Emotional | Physiological |
| *Location of change:* | Individual | Interpersonal | Community/Socio-cultural | |
| *Levels of change:* | | First order | Second order | |

### Types of change

Types of change suggests a separation between, cognition, behaviour and emotion. These are not distinct and can lead to unhelpful separations, distracting us from the recognition that all are concerned with meaning (Kelly, 1955). Behaviours and emotions are meaningful and not distinct from cognitions; all three are recursively connected so that we think, feel and act simultaneously even if our attention or focus is predominantly on one. In addition, physiological changes are a concomitant of all three of the other types of change. However, it can be helpful to use this division as a starting point for thinking about what initial position a particular therapy adopts regarding change. For example, behavioural approaches have focused their attention on behaviour, psychodynamic approaches on feelings and the cognitive therapies on cognitions. Consequently, research into the process of therapy has respectively tended to focus its attention on one or other of these types of change. More recently psychotherapy process research has also attempted to develop concepts that are pan-theoretical, such as Bordin's work on the therapeutic alliance (1979), or the assimilation model (Stiles *et al.*, 1990).

## Location of change

The second dimension, location of change, has perhaps been less clearly articulated in the psychotherapy process research literature or elsewhere. Yet this perhaps contains the most fundamental differences, not just in therapeutic approaches but also in more fundamental questions about the nature of change. Most psychotherapy research and psychotherapy process research has appeared to assume that psychotherapy is fundamentally something that is done on a one-to-one basis with an individual and their therapist. This makes the assumption that problems and human experience can be thought of as an essentially individual, intra-psychic phenomenon. As such, it runs the danger of ignoring the inter-subjective nature of human experience and of decoupling people from their cultural context. Instead, problems can be seen to arise from interpersonal contexts, family and other intimate relationships and also from the cultural expectations, demands and assumptions that professionals and others make about them.

In our experience some of the most serious and chronic cases we see are a result not of individual weakness or inadequacy but of damaging input by us, the professionals. Though we as professionals are usually attempting to be helpful, there are of course cases of the reverse, such as children in residential homes who have been abused by staff assigned to their care. There have also been extensive studies of the ways, for example, that ethnic minorities have received abusive treatment from professionals (Littlewood and Lipsedge, 1982).

## Level of change

This links to both of the above dimensions but offers a fundamental point about the level or depth of change (see also Chapter 5). It suggests that change can be 'first order', which may mean a shift in the symptoms so that they are alleviated to some extent. However, change may also be a profound change in how a person or family group see themselves, their lives and the nature of their problems (Watzlawick *et al.*, 1964, 1974). First order change can be seen in the psychoanalytic idea of symptom substitution that change may be superficial and, without a resolution of the underlying problems, may re-emerge in another form (Wollheim, 1971). Second order change, in contrast, is seen as involving a more substantial shift in emotional patterns, beliefs and relationships.

## THE SEARCH FOR THE ACTIVE INGREDIENTS OF THERAPY?

So, what is helping clients to get better? Since these therapies adopt quite different approaches, is there some underlying mechanism that is shared by all of them? Can we extract the elixir of the active ingredient of therapy? One approach that has pervaded psychotherapy research is to compare different approaches in order to illuminate what these essential ingredients might be. Coupled with an exploration of what types of problems and clients they were most effective for, this could provide an idea of what the essential differences are between different forms of psychotherapy and counselling. Unfortunately, to date, this approach has not been as helpful as it had been hoped. A large number of comparative studies have been attempted and the overall results do not suggest clear differences between the different psychotherapies (Stiles *et al.*, 1986; Bergin and Garfield, 1994; Bergin, 2003). This is despite the fact that there are major differences, or even clearly opposite positions taken, in the psychotherapies. For example, psychoanalytic approaches prescribe the use of interpretation, whereas client-centred approaches strongly exclude this, as do more recent systemic and narrative approaches. Some therapies (behavioural and psychoanalytic) generally prohibit self-disclosure by the therapist, whereas others (narrative, systemic and client-centred) utilize this. Some therapies prescribe tasks in and between sessions, for example, CBT and strategic brief therapies, while others, such as client-centred, do not usually advocate these. The many hundreds of comparative studies that have been completed have been subjected to meta-analyses which are taken to suggest little in the way of differences (Bergin and Garfield, 1994; Bergin, 2003). This has been termed the 'Dodo' effect (from *Alice in Wonderland*), where everyone wins the race and everyone gets a prize.

The picture is more complicated, however, and there have been suggestions that some of the earlier outcome studies were of low methodological quality. For example, they relied on clinically less demanding populations (such as undergraduates) and attempted to employ the therapies in less flexible manualized versions. Such manualization is a requirement in order to enable the therapies to be delivered in a standardized manner, to allow clear comparisons of the models (Stiles *et al.*, 1986).

### Fit between client and therapy

Another important point is that where differences do occur we need to be able to determine why this is the case. For example, CBT has been considered to be the therapy of choice for depression, which was seen as a form of cognitive dysfunction with an underlying tendency to misinterpret information in a negative, pessimistic manner. Though CBT has shown some good results, so have other approaches, such as interpersonal therapy and systemic (marital and family) therapies (Jones and Asen, 2000; see Chapter 5). One of the suggestions from this study was that the clients in the study were more severely depressed, hopeless, socially deprived and with previous psychiatric histories. Because systemic therapy is more able to pay attention to this complexity and the variety of contexts in which people live, it may have been more beneficial for this group than CBT, which has been found to be helpful for less severe and more recent onset groups (Jones, 2003).

Hayes *et al.* (1996) also make the important point that many studies have employed group designs in which the effects of treatments for groups have been compared. This misses out the possibility that particular treatments may be more effective for some individuals than others. For example, they suggest that clients may differ in how able they are to understand and utilize interpretations from the therapist. If the therapist attempts to 'fit' their approach to the client's needs then he or she may take more time over this and offer more interpretations so that the client learns to make use of these. However, if these clients also have more problems and are more debilitated they may still, compared to other clients, achieve relatively small improvements despite considerable input. Less debilitated clients may be able to use interpretation more effectively and make greater positive changes despite much less effort by the therapist.

Overall for the group then, it may appear that there is little correlation between the amount of interpretation offered and the amount of improvement. In fact, in order to achieve a clear statistical result, the therapist would need to be somewhat brutal and decide that it is not worth putting so much effort into more debilitated clients because the relative gains will be less. This would not be very ethical to therapists and counsellors, though it might appear to be a reasonable cost-effectiveness argument to some managers of services! However, this is something that is familiar to all psychotherapists: we know that we have to work very hard with some people and there may in fact be little change. To make our figures of effectiveness look good we would have to carefully avoid these clients or take care to refer them on to other colleagues. We leave you as readers to ponder about whether this happens in your service or not.

This suggests that psychotherapy process research needs not only to take into account client variables, which may be complex, but also to examine in detail the processes of feedback between client and therapist, such as how the therapist and client try to adjust to each other. This may require detailed case study designs (see Chapter 7).

## Specific versus common factors

A landmark in psychotherapy process research has revolved around the concept of specific as opposed to non-specific or common factors. Broadly, this is the suggestion that the lack of substantive differences between different psychotherapies comes about as a result of factors which they hold in common. More specifically, it has been suggested that the specific factors are 'technical' features, for example, exploring negative automatic thoughts in CBT, or asking circular questions in systemic family therapy. In contrast, the common factors have been seen especially to contain the interpersonal factors, such as the therapeutic relationship. There are important connections here with Carl Rogers' (1951) suggestions that there are 'facilitative conditions' created by the therapist, such as empathy, unconditional positive regard and genuineness, that are necessary and sufficient for the creation of positive therapeutic change. Strupp (1986) has argued that an unfortunate implication of this separation is the idea that the specific factors are equated to training, skill acquisition and expertise, whereas the common factors can become equated with native endowment. In effect they come to be seen as the sort of thing that anybody can do – therapy is just like having a good friend. There is a danger in this of trivializing counselling and psychotherapy and calling into question its professional legitimacy. There is also a danger in minimizing the skills that some 'good friends' possess!

However, it can be argued that the evidence does not simply indicate that specific factors are not important but that more sophisticated ways of exploring different kinds of problems may be required. Importantly, a more subtle analysis of what does take place in sessions may be required. Strupp (1986) argues that forming a positive and effective relationship with a client does in fact require a whole array of sophisticated skills. Admittedly this builds on 'natural' skills that have been acquired through life experiences outside psychotherapy training, but this does not diminish them as skills. It also builds on skills that are acquired through practice during a therapist's professional career. Therapy is seen as essentially a relationship, but one in which the therapist uses his or her personal and technical skill in every aspect of this relationship. Importantly, it addresses the issues that therapy is about building a relationship, not just about applying technical skills. He suggests four features of what these qualities may be:

1 *Formulation*. The therapist's interventions are guided by a theory which addresses the nature of the client's problems, what maintains these problems and the means for alleviating them.
2 *Reflective practice*. The therapist creates and employs an interpersonal relationship of empathy. This includes focusing on the client's needs and attending to the client's responses and communications. Throughout this, the therapist also reflects on her own needs and how these may enter into this process.
3 *Observation*. The therapist attempts to observe the client and their inter-action, understand the client's feelings, beliefs and actions, especially in terms of how these are related to their prior relationships. This under-standing involves a recognition that the effects of previous important relationships are acted out with the therapist (transference).
4 *Collaborative reformulation*. The therapist's task is to identify how feelings from previous relationships come into their relationship and to bring these to the surface and help reformulate them with the client in a way that she is able to assimilate and use.

So, to the question, 'Isn't this exactly what a good friend does?', we might answer that a good friend might be able to do many but probably not all of these.

## CONDUCTING A PSYCHOTHERAPY PROCESS RESEARCH STUDY

There are a number of key questions that arise in contemplating a piece of psychotherapy process research, as outlined in this following section.

### Whose therapy?

Research studies can be conducted on our own clinical practice or that of colleagues or other therapists (see Fig. 6.1). There are various reasons why we may chose to conduct it on our own work, as there are for exploring the work of other therapists. Conducting research into our own practice offers us direct information about what we are doing and, therefore, may be of greater relevance. It also allows us potentially deeper insights into the experiences and meaning of the therapy and into how clients experience our work with them. We can, for example, explore how our experiences as the therapist changed during the course of therapy and how these matched what our client(s) experienced.

Alternatively, researching another therapist's work can have some advantages in removing effects, such as client's wishes not to upset our feelings by mentioning less helpful aspects of their experiences with us or negative feelings that arose during therapy. Likewise, in terms of interpreting the data, it may be hard for the therapist not to be driven by powerful emotions about themselves and the clients. In some cases this may be that a therapist is overly critical of their own work if they feel they have 'failed' their client. In turn, such feelings can be a deep product of the relationship between client and therapist, for example, with a client wanting to please the therapist (and others in their life), which is a part of the problem which brought them to therapy. On the one hand, untangling such issues may be made more complex by a therapist attempting to explore their own therapy but, on the other hand, it may allow more insight than is possible by looking from the outside at another therapist's work.

Conducting research into our own practice is often more 'do-able' since we require fewer additional resources or changes to our practice. Ways of strengthening the research can include: adopting a collaborative approach, in that we share the analysis with our clients; subjecting our analysis to an independent analysis by colleagues; and conducting a form of co-research, where we mutually research our own clients and those of a colleague, and in turn he or she does the same with their own and our clients.

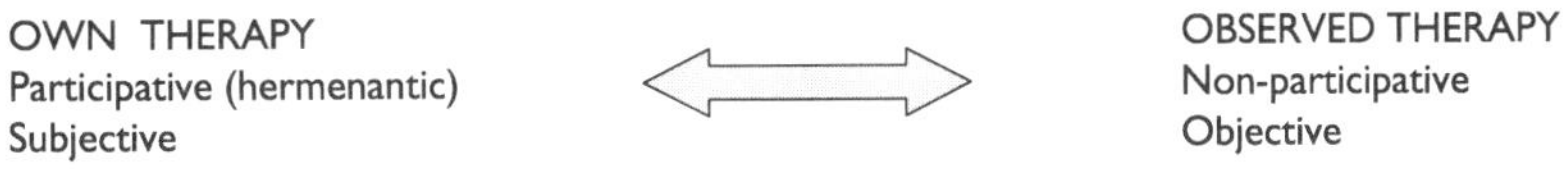

OWN THERAPY                      ⟸⟹        OBSERVED THERAPY
Participative (hermenantic)                  Non-participative
Subjective                                   Objective

**Figure 6.1**   Choice of focus of therapy process research

## General versus specific questions

The type of questions we could start with may vary in terms of how general or specific they are (see Fig. 6.2). For example, our interest may be in the nature of the experience of psychotherapy for client and therapist. Until recently many forms of psychotherapy had not been explored in terms of how they were experienced by clients. Instead, therapists had their own ideas about what was important and how change may have happened. We may want to make such exploratory studies a little more focused by inviting consideration of what was perceived as being helpful as opposed to unhelpful, when changes were seen as starting to occur and what prompted changes to occur.

In contrast, psychotherapy process studies can start with more specific and focused questions which may be attempting to test particular ideas that we hold about psychotherapy, particular client groups and problems. As an example, we might hold a hypothesis that learning to solve problems and gaining specific advice are perceived by clients to be more important in CBT therapies than emotional insights or the nature of the therapeutic relationship. These beliefs might help differentiate those who seem to benefit more, or less, from the CBT approaches.

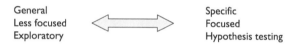

| General | | Specific |
| Less focused | | Focused |
| Exploratory | | Hypothesis testing |

**Figure 6.2** Focus of questions in therapy process research

## Meaning and actions

Research inevitably takes place in particular theoretical contexts, and in psychology, psychotherapy and counselling there has been a profound shift towards an emphasis on meaning and 'meaning-making' as central to human experience. This is in some contrast to the previous emphasis on behaviourism and behavioural interventions, though these still have a place, especially in CBT. George Kelly (1955) suggested that we should not hold a rigid distinction between actions and beliefs – both are meaningful. In our view of therapy, meaning-making and the therapeutic relationship are inextricably linked (see Fig. 6.3). The beliefs and expectations that therapists and clients bring to the encounter shape the relationship and the relationship in turn shapes the beliefs.

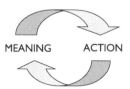

MEANING     ACTION

**Figure 6.3** Interplay of meaning and action

### Linear versus circular causality

Stiles and Shapiro (1994) have criticized the tendency in psychotherapy process research towards the use of the drug metaphor. This is the view that the active ingredients of psychotherapy can be identified by establishing correlations between various components of psychotherapy and outcome. If established this can lead to a 'more is better' dosage view of aspects of psychotherapy. Instead, they argue that psychotherapy should be thought of in terms of an iterative or systemic process, involving feedback loops (see Fig. 6.4). The therapist adjusts his or her actions according to continual feedback from the client, for example, in terms of how able they are to respond to interpretation or to different perspectives being offered. This suggests that therapy proceeds on the basis of 'moment-to-moment' adjustments to the client and, in turn, to the therapist. Methodologically it may be more difficult to capture this in terms of a linear correspondence between these factors and outcome. For example, it might be that more distressed clients may require more interpretation and work to facilitate different constructions about their lives but they may show worse overall outcomes than less distressed clients who can more easily use such interventions (Hayes *et al.*, 1996; Stiles and Shapiro, 1994).

We want to suggest that psychotherapy process research needs to include an investigation of such feedback processes. It is also possible that change for clients is associated with an experience of different ways of relating in the therapy situation. For example, an experience of sensitive and empathetic responding from another human being may be quite a new experience for many clients. In the systemic therapies the sessions invite such changes between members but also offer a new experience for a family or couple of relating to another person outside their system, for example, in less anxious, hostile or guarded ways.

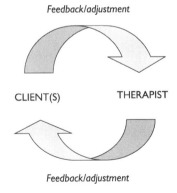

*Feedback/adjustment*

CLIENT(S)          THERAPIST

*Feedback/adjustment*

**Figure 6.4**   Therapy as a systemic/circular process of mutual adaptation between client(s) and therapist

Having outlined some criticisms of a fragmented and linear approach to research we do not want to replicate this. However, for the sake of exposition we have outlined each approach in Box 6.1 (see pp. 96–8). We invite you, however, to bear in mind connections between the approaches. For example, in thinking about the therapeutic alliance, it is clear that this embraces how a client sees not just the therapist and therapy but also themselves and, more broadly, their world view. In the next section, we focus on areas of psychotherapy process research that have been directed at the following aspects of therapy.

## EXAMPLES OF PSYCHOTHERAPY PROCESS RESEARCH STUDIES

### The therapeutic alliance

The concept of the therapeutic alliance is as old as is psychotherapy, and perhaps even older. For example, Shamanism requires a giving over of oneself to a shaman or guru. The Western precursors of therapy – the confession in Roman Catholicism – can be seen to bear important similarities to the therapeutic relationship in psychodynamic therapy giving oneself over to, trusting – God's representative on Earth – the priest. It is by working through and testing whether the therapist can react differently to 'everyone else' in one's life that the 'patient' can discover news ways of relating. Of necessity the relationship between the therapist and 'patient' will be complex, troubled and filled with strong feelings. For example, Freud (1981) suggested that his female patients inevitably fell in love with him, but not with him as a person but through a more general sense of intimacy and trust they could develop with someone: a new, fragile hope that here was someone who would not use and abuse them as others had invariably done. Further to this, his discovery of the prevalence of sexual abuse may also have had an immense emotional impact on his patients. Possibly for many, this was the first time they believed and understood about these experiences, which arguably, were denied by their friends and family. It has been suggested that such lack of acknowledgement of sexual abuse was a feature of the attitudes prevalent in 'respectable' Viennese society at that time.

The concept of the therapeutic alliance has been elaborated by Bordin (1979) to embrace all forms of psychotherapy. In addition to the emotional bonding with the therapist, he suggests that there is an agreement on the goals of the therapy and the tasks this will involve:

- *Therapeutic bond*. This is the client's overall positive affectional bond with the therapist and includes their sense of trust, belief in the therapist's abilities, positive expectations of help from the therapist, collaboration and involvement.
- *Therapeutic goals*. Explicit contract which includes clarity and agreement of overall goals, ways to achieve these and how to monitor progress.
- *Therapeutic tasks*. Clarity and agreement on the tasks of therapy, including ground rules, responsibilities, mutual roles and consent.

According to Leiper (2001), research indicates that how the relationship starts – the initial strength of the alliance – is one of the best predictors of eventual outcome (Horvath and Symonds, 1991). Failure to develop a good relationship is very likely to lead to drop-out from treatment. As therapy may be difficult and painful at times, it requires a strong therapeutic alliance to assist the client through these times – to keep hope and faith to persevere.

Research Example 6.1 outlines a study of the therapeutic alliance and therapeutic outcome.

---

**Research Example 6.1**

Luborsky, L., Critis-Cristoph, P., Leslie-Alexander, M. S., Margolis, M. and Cohen, M. (1983) Two helping alliance methods for predicting outcome of psychotherapy, *Journal of Nervous and Mental Disease*, 171(8): 480–91.

Luborsky and his colleagues define the therapeutic alliance in terms of a 'helping alliance' and 'the person's experience of the treatment or the relationship with the therapist as helpful, or potentially helpful, in achieving their goals'. Further, the alliance is seen to fall into two types:

- Type 1 – the therapist is experienced as *providing*, or being capable of providing, the help which is needed.
- Type 2 – the treatment is experienced more as *working together* with the therapist towards the goals of treatment.

*Aims and questions*: To explore the validity of the two types above, to examine whether the alliance could predict outcome of psychotherapy and to explore the validity of their alliance coding system.

*Design and method*: Twenty participants were selected from 73 who had taken part in 'supportive-expressive psychoanalytically oriented psychotherapy', delivered by 18 psychiatrists of varying experience. The participants were divided into two groups: High improvement – the ten most improved; and Low improvement – the ten least improved. The improvement was based on two measures: overall improvement and pre–post therapy differences. The first 20 minutes were transcribed from sessions 3 and 5 and two late sessions. All patients had at least 25 one-hour sessions.

*Sample*: The 20 participants were attending a psychiatric outpatient clinic in the USA. They were non-psychotic, 15 were female, the mean age was 26 and the demographic characteristics of the High and Low improvement groups were similar.

*Measure and analysis*: A scoring manual was developed which required the identification of episodes in transcripts indicating alliance types 1 or 2. Each of the subtypes could be scored positively or negatively: for example, if the client appeared to be suggesting that the therapy was *not* helping and was rated from 1 (very low) to 5 (very high). The transcripts were analysed by two independent trained raters (both experienced psychoanalysts), giving agreements of 0.82.

*Results*: Significant differences were found between the High and Low improvement group. The high group showed much higher positive helping alliance scores in the early sessions and this increased considerably as therapy progressed, whereas for the Low group the reverse was the case. This further indicated an escalating process in the therapy of either enhancement or deterioration of the helping alliance. The two alliance types were found to be highly correlated.

## Exploring the experience of psychotherapy: constructivist approaches

The starting position for this approach is rooted in qualitative research that aims to explore psychotherapy by attempting to map the phenomenology or experience of psychotherapy from the participant's perspective. One of the major contributors to this approach has been David Rennie (1992) and his colleagues in the Department of Psychology at York University in Toronto (Canada), where they have conducted a series of studies exploring the clients' experiences of psychotherapy (see Research Example 6.2). His approach is based in a constructivist approach which regards clients and therapists as mutually engaging in a process of meaning-making. Furthermore, it adopts the view that clients are able to reflect and comment on their experiences and research, as therapy can be a collaborative activity rather than an expert doing things to, or needing to interpret the experience for the client. This approach adds an important twist to qualitative research in that it fully accepts the client and therapist as active collaborators in the research by placing their ability to reflect on their experience as central.

### Research Example 6.2

Rennie, D. (1992) Qualitative analysis of the client's experience of psychotherapy: the unfolding of reflexivity, in S. C. Toukmanis and D. Rennie (eds) *Psychotherapy Process Research: Paradigmatic and Narrative Approaches*. London: Sage.

*Aims and questions*: The study attempted to gain an 'inside' view from clients of their experience of psychotherapy, including what was perceived to be important and helpful as opposed to unhelpful. Rather than imposing 'a priori' hypotheses or categories, a 'grounded theory' was employed which derived themes, grounded in the client's accounts (Glaser and Strauss, 1967).

*Design*: The study employed exploratory open-ended interviews with 14 clients attending counselling services. Participants were included on the basis of having relatively non-acute problems (non-psychotic) and all had a good enough relationship with their therapist to 'handle such a sensitive research endeavour'.

*Method*: The interviews were conducted by two colleagues who interviewed each other's clients, immediately after a therapy session. The clients had been in therapy for various lengths of time, ranging from six weeks to more than two years. The 11 therapists (six men and five women) all had over five years' experience as therapists: five were person-centred, two Gestalt, one rational–emotive, one radical behaviourist/person-centred and one transactional/analytic/Gestalt.

The interviews were facilitated by the method of 'interpersonal process recall' in which the interviewer replays the tape of the session to assist the participant's recall (see Chapter 9). Clients were invited to stop the tape when they felt anything significant was happening, though on occasion the therapist initiated discussion if participants passed over substantial segments of tape. The interviews lasted from two to four hours and were transcribed giving from 40 to 80 pages of material.

*Sample*: The clients were six men, and eight women who were attending university and private counselling services.

*Analysis*: A grounded theory analysis was employed (see Chapter 4).

*Findings*: The analysis produced four main themes, with the first found to be the most frequent:

- The client's relationship with personal meanings
- The client's perception of the relationship with the therapist
- The client's experience of the therapist's operations
- The client's experience of outcomes.

Overall the study revealed a core theme of 'reflexivity' or self-awareness. The accounts were seen to show that clients were thinking in insightful and complex ways about the therapy in terms of their own feelings, what was right for them and in what ways they needed to control the process of therapy.

Rennie noted that much of such thinking processes had not been evident to the therapists. He argued that such research invites clients' reflexivity and that the content of this may be missed by research which simply looks at the dialogue of therapy sessions. By inviting clients to become co-researchers insight can be gained into the sophistication and complexity of their understandings during the process of therapy.

The next study explored the experience of a less verbally sophisticated group, namely children's experiences of family therapy (see Research Example 6.3). Despite the fact that one of the most common applications of family therapy has been in relation to children's problems, there has been little research on how children experience therapy and what this might tell us about ways of making the process interesting and effective for them.

### Research Example 6.3

Stith, S. M., Rosen, K. H., McCollum, E. E., Coleman, J. U. and Herman, S. A. (1996) The voices of children: preadolescent children's experiences in family therapy, *Journal of Marital and Family Therapy*, 22: 69–86.

This study involved 16 children (aged between 5 and 12) undergoing therapy with their families (12 families in total). Fourteen of the children were white and two were Afro-American; ten of the children were in single-parent families (headed by single mothers), four were in nuclear families, one was in a remarried family and one child was being raised by grandparents. Eleven of the 12 families presented with child-focused problems and the remaining family identified marital problems as the main concern.

Therapists were asked to invite families to participate and the families were then contacted by a researcher. Children were usually interviewed while the parents were seeing the therapist. Each child was interviewed twice and the parents were interviewed once.

*Method*: A semi-structured interview lasting about half an hour was employed. Children were invited to tell their experience of therapy in their own words, but a number of general questions were included, such as: 'When you and your family talk about coming here, what do you call this place?', 'What happens when you and your family come here?', 'What do you like/don't like about coming here?') 'Do you ever wonder about the people behind the mirror?', 'What do you think about them?'

An attempt was made to compare the children's accounts with their parent's or a teenage sibling's perceptions of the child's experience. These interviews employed a number of questions, such as: 'What do you think (e.g. Mary) thinks about coming to family therapy?', 'How does he or she respond when it's time to come to therapy?'

*Analysis and results*: The interviews were transcribed and members of the team then independently analysed two of the initial transcripts employing a 'grounded theory' framework. The children's experiences were found to group into four areas or themes:

1 The reactions of the children to the process of video-taping and live supervision.
2 How they understood why they and their families had come to therapy.
3 How they described what happened in therapy.
4 What they said had changed during the time they had been coming to therapy.

In general, all the children interviewed indicated a desire to be included actively in the therapy. All but the youngest understood the purpose of therapy and reported that talking about problems was helpful to them and their families. The younger children (aged 5–9) enjoyed play activities and believed the personality of the therapist to be important. One of the key findings was that children wished to be included but did not wish to be the sole focus. They wanted to learn more about the workings of their family, help in the solutions of problems and not have their own troubles as the focus. The responses of the parents and siblings also suggested that children were more comfortable the more they knew about the reasons the family had come for therapy. Though initially resistant, the children saw some value in the sessions over time. Finally, the researchers suggested that therapists who are interested in children, able to express warmth and connection to them and willing to operate in the child's world will have more success involving them in therapy.

Research Example 6.4 outlines a study using repertory grids to explore changes in beliefs, expectations and construings in the course of therapy.

### Research Example 6.4

Ben Tovim, D. I. and Greenup, J. (1983) The representation of the transference relationship through serial grids: a methodological study, *British Journal of Medicinal Psychology*, 56: 255–62.

This study employed repertory grids (see Chapter 5) to map changes in a client's perceptions regarding her relationship with her therapist and other significant people in her life during the course of therapy. Specifically, one of the intentions of the study was to explore changes in the therapeutic relationship and to consider these in terms of transference. This was defined as the extent to which the relationship with the therapist was seen as similar to other important relationships in the client's life, for example, the similarities of her construing of her relationship with her mother and father and that between herself and her therapist.

*Method*: A repertory grid was administered following each of 13 sessions of psychotherapy. This consisted of 22 elements, including the following:

Me now with my father
Me with my father when I was a
  child
Me now with my therapist
Me with my mother when I was a child
Me with my mother now
Ideal self with therapist
Mother with father
Past boyfriend with me
etc.

My father now with me
My father with me when I was
  a child
My therapist with me now
My mother with me as a child
My mother with me now
Therapist with my ideal self
Father with mother
Me with past boyfriend

Using these elements, 11 constructs were elicited, such as rational–emotional, kind–unkind, aggressive–nonaggressive, reliable–unreliable. The same grids were employed at the end of each session (new constructs were not elicited on each occasion).

All sessions were recorded and transcribed and subjected to an analysis in terms of the therapist's interventions. These were classified in terms of general, empathetic, questions, reassurance and interpretations.

*Results*: A form of correlation was attempted of the 'distances' between pairs of relationships. Changes in the perceived similarity over the sessions indicated changes in the possible transference relationships (see below Fig. 6.5). This shows changes in the client's perceptions regarding her relationship with her father when she was a child and her current relationship with her therapist.

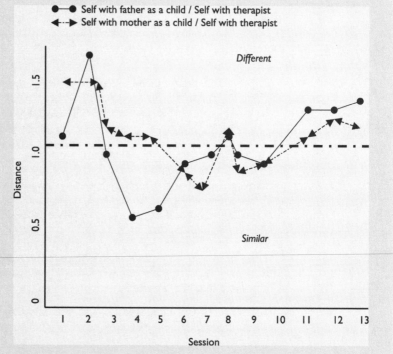

**Figure 6.5**   Changes in client's perceptions of her relationship with self as a child and her father and her current relationship with her therapist

Changes in the similarities between various relationships were mapped. Figure 6.5 indicates that the client in the first sessions saw her relationship with her therapist as different to her relationship with her father and mother when she was a child. However, as therapy progresses it appears that she started to see these two relationships as more similar, especially in the third and fourth sessions where she appeared to see similarity between her relationship with her therapist and her relationship with her father when she was a child. In session 6 and 7 it appears that she started to see less similarity between these two relationships and moved to seeing a closer similarity between her relationship as a child with her mother and her relationship with her therapist.

This offers a picture of the development and changes in transferences as therapy progresses. It suggests that early in therapy she saw the relationship with her therapist as similar to her relationship as a child to her father. A little later this moves towards seeing more of a similarity to the relationship with her mother. As therapy proceeds she gradually came to differentiate the relationships with her therapist to her childhood relationship with her father and mother. This seems to indicate that she had started to differentiate these relationships and that there was less of a transference from these important early relationships involved in her relationship with her therapist. The grids also allowed a similar analysis of fluctuations in such comparisons regarding a range of relationships. This interestingly offers a much broader picture of transference as involving the application of construings from a range of relationships.

The study also allowed an analysis of how particular types of interventions appeared to influence changes in construings. These indicated that for this client the only significant effects were that interpretations from the therapist specifically about her relationship with her father, or interpretations naming her father, did produce changes two weeks later in her construing of her relationship with him.

Winter (2003) makes the point that repertory grid techniques are eminently suited for psychotherapy process research in that they can capture the uniqueness of therapy process and also offer a means for developing quantitative exploration. Like personal questionnaires (which can in fact be seen as a form of repertory grid), they are a good example of the potential of mixed methods in psychotherapy research.

## Significant events research

This research has roots in many therapeutic traditions and also has employed a variety of research methods. Studies start from the premise that change in psychotherapy is punctuated by significant or key events. This idea is further based on the premise that all therapies are concerned with helping clients assimilate problematic experiences:

> First, all therapies offer a forum in which prolonged attention can be brought to bear on painful or puzzling experience. Second, all involve the elaboration of coherent schemata – frameworks in which the problematic experiences can be understood.
>
> (Stiles *et al.*, 1990, p. 416)

It is argued that for clients, especially those with more severe problems, their schemas or frames of understanding are unable to take in or assimilate difficult experiences of hurt, shame and failure. For example, they may be avoided, suppressed or denied because they are too threatening to self-esteem. Such experiences are partly in our awareness and attempts to make sense of them can be painful and distressing. Drawing on Piagetian concepts of assimilation and accommodation, Stiles suggests that *assimilation* is the process whereby experiences are taken in, integrated and made sense of (see Fig. 6.6). This requires a shift in the person's schema. In this process experiences are also *accommodated*, which involves some change in how the experience is seen. Shifts in both are required for therapeutic change to occur. For example, accommodation alone can involve attempts to distort an event so that it fits within our schemas or beliefs about ourself.

The assimilation model suggests that therapy can be seen to start at various points along the continuum. For severe problems early in the assimilation process, the experiences may be warded off and not available for contemplation. Later they become available but are painful so that clients have limited capacity to endure the distress that may be reactivated. Later on in the process they may be felt as problematic, puzzling and

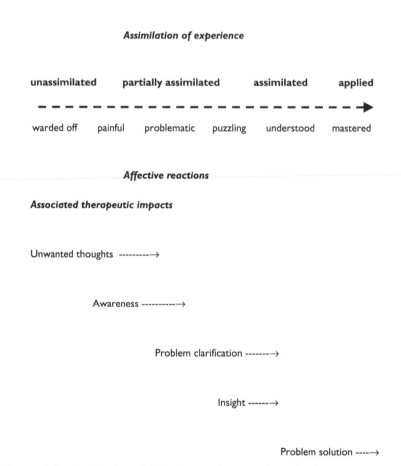

**Figure 6.6**  Assimilation of difficult experiences and psychotherapy
From: Stiles, *et al.* 1990, p. 413.

eventually become understood and accepted with a sense of confidence. Specifically, it is suggested that:

> Although assimilation can occur gradually, inside or outside therapy sessions, some events within therapy sessions produce sudden, dramatic increases in assimilation . . . (and) give rise to strong affective reactions.
>
> (Stiles *et al.*, 1990, p. 414)

The concept of assimilation also connects with ideas about the importance of ruptures in the therapeutic relationship drawn from research on the therapeutic alliance. Safran *et al.* (1990) likewise suggest that helping to change a client's unhelpful schemas is central to therapy. They add that clients may unconsciously test their therapist to see if they will respond in the ways that they expect to be treated on the basis of their previous experience. So, for example, a client who anticipates that others will attempt to dominate her may act in a passive, apathetic way which invites the therapist to take charge, thus confirming her belief that this will always be the case for her and causing her to withdraw further. This can lead to a 'rupture' in the alliance, in that both clients and therapist may feel bad, let down, angry and frustrated with each other. Safran *et al.* suggest that it is at these points that 'significant events' or change can occur if this rupture is addressed. This connects with Stiles *et al.*'s (1990) discussion above of the extent to which significant events tend to be emotionally laden: both client and therapist often feel more awake, connected and excited, especially when changes in the schemas become possible.

A study into significant events in psychotherapy is outlined in Research Example 6.5.

---

**Research Example 6.5**

Llewelyn, S. P., Elliot, R., Shapiro, D. A., Hardy, G. and Firth-Cozens, J. (1988) Client perceptions of significant events in prescriptive and exploratory periods of individual therapy, *British Journal of Clinical Psychology*, 27: 105–14.

Llewelyn *et al.* attempted to explore the views of clients concerning the most helpful and unhelpful events that they perceived to have occurred in exploratory versus prescriptive therapies.

*Design*: A comparative, cross-over design was employed in which 40 clients received eight sessions of exploratory (psychodynamic/verbal) and eight sessions of prescriptive (cognitive behavioural) therapy. Each client received therapy from the same therapist and the order of the therapies was counterbalanced so that half the sample received exploratory therapy first and the other half prescriptive first. The treatments were manualized.

*Sample*: The 40 clients were referred by their GP for therapy for depression and/or anxiety – none were psychotic. All of them were professional or managerial staff.

*Measures*: At the end of each therapy session clients completed the Helpful Aspects of Therapy (HAT) Questionnaire, which asked for descriptions of the most helpful event that had occurred, as well as any other event including negative ones. Similarly, they were asked to describe their experience at the end of both eight-session forms of therapy.

A variety of outcome measures were employed: the Present State Examination, the Symptom Checklist and also the Beck Depression Inventory, Social Adjustment Scale and Rosenberg Self-Esteem scale.

*Analysis*: The descriptions provided in the questionnaires were subjected to a content analysis by three independent raters which employed 14 categories derived from the work of Elliott (1984). These included positive categories – personal insight, awareness, problem solution, problem clarification, involvement, understanding, reassurance, personal contact – and negative categories – unwanted thoughts, unwanted responsibility, misdirection and repetition. Inter-rater reliability was reasonably high, at between 0.85 and 0.55.

*Results*: The analysis was based on frequencies of events and this showed that clients saw the most commonly occurring impacts as 'awareness' and 'problem solution' for the prescriptive therapy and 'awareness' and 'personal insight' for the exploratory therapy. This was consistent with the aims of the two types of therapy. The prescriptive therapy gained significantly more negative evaluations: unwanted thoughts, repetition and misdirection. These effects were replicated for the two types of therapy overall.

However, there was no significant relationship between the frequencies reported of the helpful events and outcome. The researchers commented that frequencies may not capture the meaning or quality of significant helpful events. They suggested a need for a finer differentiation of the events by using a rating scale of the impact of each event. Also, they suggested it is important to employ a more qualitative case study approach to examine the meaning of events in therapy sessions.

## Systemic/process studies: what therapists actually 'do' in sessions

A number of researchers have conducted observational studies to explore what happens in psychotherapy sessions. This is a relatively recent development, at least for some therapies, such as psychoanalytic therapies, which regarded therapy as necessarily a 'closed' private experience. It was felt that observation or recording of sessions could damage the therapeutic relationship. We might note that, of course, therapists are always engaged in observation, for example, a client's expressions, posture, reactions and synchronization with their actions. In addition, therapists try to observe their own actions and reactions, though clearly this is often hard to do. Early studies indicated, for example, that therapists were often engaging in a wide range of behaviour, of which they were not only unaware but which, in some cases, was quite inconsistent with the theory underlying the therapy.

One of the earliest and most famous studies was conducted by Truax (1966) to examine Rogerian psychotherapy through a behavioural lens (see Research Example 6.6). As such, it was one of the first attempts to challenge the premises on which a psychotherapy was based by looking at what happens in action to examine whether an alternative explanation for its effects is more plausible.

---

**Research Example 6.6**

Truax, C. B. (1966) Reinforcement and non-reinforcement in Rogerian Psychotherapy, *Journal of Abnormal Psychology*, 71(1): 1–9.

In this study, video recordings were made of Rogerian counselling sessions. In these the counsellor takes an exploratory and non-directive approach which aims to encourage an active position on the part of the client, including them in decisions on the direction, goal, tasks and techniques of therapy.

*Design*: A single, long-term successful therapy case handled by Rogers was examined.

*Method*: Tape recordings of the 85 sessions were made and 20 of these (at regular intervals over the sessions) were employed for analysis. Two interaction units were employed. These were the first third and the second third of each sessions. Each section of the session was transcribed. These consisted of statements by the therapist, responses by the client and responses to this from the therapist. Five clinical psychologists independently rated extracts from the transcripts.

*Analysis*: The extracts were analysed in terms of:

- coding the therapists responses to the client's statements – empathetic understanding, acceptance or unconditional positive regard and directiveness.
- coding the client's statements – degree of learning of discriminations, ambiguity, insight, similarity in style of expression to the therapist's, degree of anxiety, blocking positive versus negative expressions, catharsis.

*Results*: The qualitative analysis revealed that Rogers' style was to restate what the client had said, avoid psychological jargon and use tentative phrases, such as 'in a sense', 'I guess' and 'maybe'. Correlations based on ratings of the therapist and client codes above revealed significant links between the client's statements and how Rogers responded. For example, where the client showed insight or spoke in a similar manner to the therapist this resulted in responses of empathy and acceptance from Rogers. Furthermore, it appeared that, as a consequence, these behaviours increased over the course of the therapy.

Rogers was highly committed to psychotherapy research. He was one of the first psychotherapists to record his sessions and to expose his work to close scrutiny. For example, the study detailed in Research Example 6.6 comes from a series of studies in collaboration with Truax, despite this research clearly questioning some of Rogers' core assumptions (Rogers and Truax, 1965).

The study outlined in Research Example 6.7 likewise employed an analysis of transcripts from therapy sessions to explore the conversational actions in narrative therapy with families.

### Research Example 6.7

Coulehan, R., Friedlander, M. L. and Heatherington, L. (1988) Transforming narratives: a change event in constructivist family therapy, *Family Process*, 37: 17–33.

The study was framed within a version of narrative therapy which emphasizes that the process of change involves transformations of negative stories surrounding the presenting problem.

*Aims:* The study was an attempt to examine the actions of therapists and responses of clients that led to successful transformations. The study also aimed to explore the idea that transformation occurs through a shift in an initial story which typically focuses on intra-psychic explanations and person blaming, followed by creating a new interpersonally focused story.

*Design:* The study employed a structural analysis of therapist–family conversations in 8 sessions of narrative therapy with 8 different families. A comparative design was employed in which four families, where the session had produced a shift in the family members' view of the presenting problem, were compared with four where there had been no such shift.

*Sample:* Eight families took part in the study with a child focused referral: two intact, one remarried, four single-parent families and one headed by a grandparent. Multiple problems were described including verbal abusiveness, non-compliance, compulsive overeating, school failure and other behavioural difficulties. Several of the children were or had been in foster homes or residential settings. The overall treatment ranged from 2 to 12 sessions and was not different for the two family groups.

The therapists (four women and four men) had an age range of 28–59. Two were psychologists, one a psychiatrist and one had a Masters degree level qualification in therapy or counselling. All were trained in Sluzki's narrative family therapy approach.

*Method:* The study consisted of analysis of video-tapes of the first session of therapy with eight families. The therapists all attempted to facilitate a transformation of the problem. In four sessions the transformation was independently judged to be successful by the therapist and observers, whilst in four other sessions the transformation was judged to be unsuccessful. The sessions were video-taped and subsequently transcribed.

*Analysis*: The therapists indicated immediately after the session whether they felt a successful transition had occurred. The video-tapes were repeatedly viewed by independent raters and following a discussion a consensus was reached regarding successful transformation or otherwise in the session. Unfortunately, the questionnaire used to gain the family's evaluation of the sessions was found to be unsatisfactory.

The Cognitive Constructions Coding System was employed. The transcript was broken into episodes which contained a discussion of the problems. Within each episode occurrences of explanations were noted in terms of intra-personal–interpersonal dimension. The order of speaking turns was noted, as were tactics employed by the therapist, and note was also made of the emotional reactions in the sessions.

*Results*: The four families for whom the initial sessions were seen to contain transformations reported positive changes. In the four where the initial session did not, two later reported some positive changes but two dropped out from treatment.

The findings added support to Sluzki's (1992) notion of change but elaborated it into a three-stage model:

1 Families expressing their initial views of the problems, followed by a discussion of relevant interpersonal dynamics and exceptions to the problems, were encouraged.
2 A move towards positive attributions and family strengths was encouraged and the therapist blocked attempts at a return to blaming. There was a detectable shift in the families' emotional tone.
3 Hope or possibility of change was acknowledged, with a shift in the emotional tone from blaming to a more nurturant supportive position.

The study also revealed that the therapists inspired hope in the family (connecting with the idea of establishing a good alliance). Also the therapists were active and in some cases directive, for example, blocking negative and blaming conversations. Finally, it was clear that therapy involved an important emotional component within which the therapist was able to connect and nurture.

## Client and therapist variables

A range of studies have employed an examination of particular aspects of therapy process in terms of the interactions between therapist's actions and client factors.

Smith (1996) argues forcefully that inadequate attention has been paid to the fact that therapists differ in their effectiveness in relation to different types of clients and problems. An exploration of these differences can also point up what may be the active components of psychotherapy. A number of factors were identified in a study by Blatt *et al.* (1996), outlined in Research Example 6.8.

**Research Example 6.8**

Blatt, J. S., Sanislow III, C. A., Zuroff, D. C. and Pilkonins, P. A. (1996) Characteristics of effective therapists: further analysis from the National Institute of Mental Health Treatment of Depression and Collaborative Research Programme, *Journal of Consulting and Clinical Psychology*, 64(6): 1276–84.

The study consisted of an examination of the performance of 28 therapists who were treating clients for depression as part of the above programme. This is a comprehensive randomized clinical control trial which has been exploring outpatient treatment for depression. The therapies employed consisted of CBT, interpersonal psychotherapy or medication.

*Aims*: These were to attempt to identify factors amongst the therapists that were linked to successful treatment.

*Method*: The 28 therapists treated between three and nine patients. The therapists were of equivalent professional standing with an average of 11 years of clinical experience; the male–female ratio was 20:8. A range of measures (five) were employed, including the BDI and SCL-90 to assess change in their clients. These were subjected to factor analysis to reveal one dominant factor of effectiveness. Demographic details were collected for each therapist and they completed a questionnaire concerned with explanations of depression, use of medication, their expectations of success and ideas about what produced change.

*Analysis*: The therapists were split into three groups: high, medium and low 'effectives'. The therapists' variables and attitudes were compared for the three groups.

*Results*: Effectiveness was not related to the types of therapy employed nor to the level of general clinical experience or experience of treating depression. More effective therapists had a more psychological rather than physiological orientation; they almost invariably used psychotherapy on its own with clients and very rarely employed medical interventions. They were also more likely to be psychologists than psychiatrists. There were no clear differences in attitudes to depression and its causes, with the exception that the more effective therapists felt that more sessions were necessary before any change could start to be shown.

This study connects with other findings that a therapist's beliefs in a treatment may be communicated either explicitly or implicitly to clients. In the study the belief in psychotherapy and the disinclination to use medication perhaps most clearly identifies a therapist's commitment to, and belief in, the value of psychotherapy for their clients with depression.

A study by Patterson and Forgatch (1985), detailed in Research Example 6.9, explores another important therapist and client variable, namely the issue of compliance and non-compliance. For therapy to progress, there needs to be agreement and an element of working together, and it is important to explore what aspects of the therapist's behaviour may serve to increase or decrease compliance and cooperation.

### Research Example 6.9

Patterson, G. R. and Forgatch, M. S. (1985) Therapist behaviour as a determinant for client non-compliance: a paradox for the behaviour modifier, *Journal of Consulting and Clinical Psychology*, 53(6): 846–51.

This study was an attempt to explore an important issue in psychotherapy which relates to the working alliance, namely compliance or non-compliance. Many therapists experience that certain attempts to assist clients, such as giving advice, teaching and confronting, may stimulate the client to work against rather than with the therapist. In this particular study, the approach was 'parent training' – an approach which is used extensively in the context of work with young offenders. It is also an approach which notoriously attracts resistance from families who may feel patronized or 'told off'.

*Aims*: The study attempted to examine through observation of therapy sessions how non-compliance occurred. The intention was to examine both the actions of the therapist and clients' response to this. Two studies were conducted to examine the relationships between therapist and client reactions and also to explore the causal relationship between them.

*Design*: Two related studies were conducted. In the first, the therapy with six families was video-taped and the sequence of actions of the therapist and reactions of the family were analysed. In the second study, a reversal ABAB design was employed in which the therapist engaged in 'teach' and 'confront' activities in phase A and attempted to reduce these in phase B.

*Sample*: In study 1, there were six families with child management problems – five social aggression and one chronically delinquent. Half the families had an absent father. The five therapists (four female, one male) were experienced (2–15 years). In study 2, there were seven families – four social aggression and three child abuse (four girls and three boys; mean age 7.8). Five had an absent father and the families were relatively economically poor.

*Method*: In study 1, the therapy consisted of 20 hours of work. Only the mothers' behaviour was employed in the study. The mothers' and the therapists' behaviours were scored independently from video-tapes of the sessions. Initially client behaviour was scored using the Client Non-compliance Code. Following this an independent rater coded the therapist behaviour using the Therapist Behaviour Code.

   Study 2 employed a similar form of analysis, but the therapist changed their behaviour from an emphasis on teaching and confrontation in period A to a more exploratory approach in period B. This was then repeated.

*Analysis*: The analysis was based on the conditional probabilities of therapist–client behaviours. Client non-compliance behaviours were coded in terms of: interrupt, negative attitude, confront, own agenda, not tracking. One category described all compliant behaviour. Therapist behaviour was classified in terms of: support, teach, question, confront, reframe, talk and facilitate. The video-tapes were coded independently, with 0.65 per cent agreement.

*Results*: Study 1 revealed that the actions of 'teaching' and 'confrontation' were significantly likely to be immediately followed by a range of non-compliance behaviours by the mothers. In contrast, the actions 'facilitate' and 'support' were likely to produce a significant decrease in the probability of non-compliance behaviours.

Study 2 indicated a clear link, such that as the therapist increased their behaviour of 'teach' and 'confront' client non-compliance rose significantly and when they reduced their 'teach' and 'confront' behaviour client non-compliance reduced to baseline level. However, non-compliance decreased in the second B period (despite a decrease in teach/confront).

The authors point out that the studies suggest that therapists, in the face of non-compliance, may come to view the family in a negative way, become distant and give up on the family. The findings that 'support' and 'facilitate' increased compliance suggest ways that compliance can be fostered.

This study is a good example of an attempt to address some of the criticisms offered by Davey (2003) regarding clinical research. The first study outlined in Research Example 6.8 offers a correlational analysis of the relationship between therapist actions and client non-compliance. However, the study in Research Example 6.9 develops this to explore the causal connection between therapist behaviour and client non-compliance by an experimental reversal ABAB design. This helps to offer evidence of a convincing causal connection.

## Interpersonal models of change

These studies connect with the research on the therapeutic alliance in proposing that therapy occurs as a consequence of a new type of interpersonal experience in therapy. Specifically, it is suggested that the therapeutic relationship can offer a new way of relating that offers an opportunity for the client to change:

individuals come to treat themselves as they have been treated by others . . . the therapist's interpersonal behaviour towards the patient would either serve to entrench a negative introject or be sufficiently different and consistent to allow for ameliorative re-introjection and introject change.

(Hilliard *et al.*, 2000, p. 125)

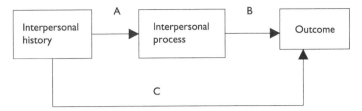

**Figure 6.7**   Psychotherapy and the influence of clients' and therapists' personal histories

A summary of the model is offered (see Fig. 6.7 and Research Example 6.10). This suggests that clients' and therapists' histories can be seen to influence the outcome both directly and also through its influence on the interpersonal process in therapy (A and B). In turn, the interpersonal process, or therapeutic relationship, can shape outcome (C).

---

**Research Example 6.10**

Hilliard, R. B., Henry, W. P. and Strupp, H. H. (2000) An interpersonal model of psychotherapy: linking patient and therapist developmental history, therapeutic process and type of outcome, *Journal of Consulting and Clinical Psychology*, 68(1): 125–33.

This study attempted to explore an interpersonal model of therapy and particularly the idea that the effect of the client's personal history mediated, and was mediated by, the therapeutic relationship.

*Aims*: The study aimed to explore how clients' and therapists' interpersonal histories shaped the process of therapy and outcome. As part of this, the study attempted to develop a sophisticated way of describing the therapeutic process in interpersonal terms.

*Design*: A correlational design was employed to examine the relationship between early parental relationships of clients and therapists and how these correlated with process in the third session of therapy and overall outcome.

*Sample*: Fifty clients (77 per cent women) of diverse backgrounds, problems and prior experience of therapy. Sixteen therapists took part, ten of which were men. There were eight psychologists and six psychiatrists.

*Method*: The therapists were observed in their third session with two clients. It was felt that the quality of the therapeutic relationship would be well established by this time. An average 21.4 weekly sessions were conducted.

*Measures*: Early parental relationships for clients and therapists were assessed through the SASB INTREX questionnaire, which provided a measure of the quality of the relationship to each parent.

Outcomes were measured by changes from intake to termination of therapy, assessed by: the SASB INTROJECT questionnaire, which assesses self-perception and acceptance of self, symptoms by the SCK-90 (Derogatis), GOR (Global Outcome Rating) scale.

*Analysis*: A detailed analysis, using the SASB coding system (Benjamin, 1974) was undertaken in the third session, which was video-taped and analysed independently by two sets of coders and by means of a questionnaire by the therapist and client. The focus was on the nature of the 'affiliation' between the therapists and clients. Analysis employed repeated viewing of the video-tape with accompanying analysis of the transcript.

*Results*: Regression analyses indicated that the clients' early parental relationships had a direct effect on outcome and a mediational effect on outcome, mediated through the effect on therapy process. Also, it was found that therapists' early relations directly influenced outcome and therapy process, despite their extensive training in psychotherapy which attempts to address the influence of their family histories.

### Cycle of change research and choice of therapeutic approach

A commonly reported observation across a wide variety of therapies is that clients appear to have different levels of motivation or intention of changing (see also Howard *et al.* in Chapter 5). In psychodynamic therapies this was described as 'resistance', in others as fear of change and in systemic therapies as 'homeostasis' or inertia in the family system. Prochaska and DiClemente (1982, 1992) developed these ideas to suggest that clients can be regarded as being at different stages of readiness to change. They suggest that this is a transtheoretical model, in that the stages that they have identified apply to all therapies and, importantly, can be used to guide the choice of therapy, or therapeutic emphasis, for clients at different stages. An important argument they offer is that often lack of progress in therapy occurs due to lack of attention to where the client is in terms of their readiness to change.

Prochaska and DiClemente understand their model of change to be spiral, in that people may well progress through contemplation, preparation and action but most will relapse and return to earlier stages in the model (see Fig. 6.8).

Some may return to pre-contemplation and give up any hope of changing. However, the spiral model suggests that people do not endlessly go round in circles, but rather that each time they relapse they have an opportunity to learn from their efforts and mistakes and to try something in a different way next time. Thus the need to assess a person's readiness to change and tailor interventions accordingly is apparent. Prochaska and DiClemente's cycle of change model is outlined in Research Example 6.11.

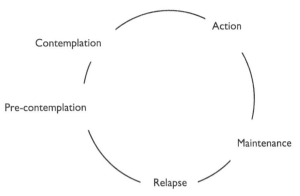

**Figure 6.8**    Cycle of change model of psychotherapy

**Research Example 6.11**

Prochaska, J. O. and DiClemente, C. C. (1982) Transtheoretical therapy: towards a more integrative model of change, *Psychotherapy; Theory, Research and Practice*, 20: 161–73.

Based on observation of therapy and an overview of the literature, Prochaska and DiClemente developed a hypothetical framework which considered change to occur through a number of relatively discrete stages. In order to explore this model they employed two different self-report measures:

1 A discrete categorical measure which assesses the stages of change from a series of mutually exclusive questions.
2 A continuous measure which yielded separate scales for the stages of change.

This model was employed in the context of a variety of psychological problems but particularly in relation to addictive disorders, such as smoking, drug addiction and eating problems.

Prochaska and DiClemente examined the processes involved in change. Through the use of self-report instruments and transcriptions of psychotherapy sessions, they identified ten different processes. When the stages of change were matched to the processes of change, they found typical patterns that have implications for the most appropriate forms of therapy for each stage. Below is a summary of the processes that increased at each stage:

- *Pre-contemplations*: less use of any of the processes
- *Contemplation*: consciousness-raising, emotional arousal, environmental re-evaluation
- *Contemplation*: self-re-evaluation
- *Preparation*: self-liberation

■ *Action*: Reward, helping relationships, counter-conditioning and environmental control.

In summary, Prochaska and DiClemente argue that different types of therapy may be suitable according to the stage of change of each client:

change processes traditionally associated with the experiential, cognitive, and psychodynamic persuasions are most useful during the pre-contemplation and contemplation stages. Change processes associated with the existential and behavioural traditions, by contrast, are most useful during action and maintenance.

(Prochaska *et al.*, 1992, p. 1112)

Interestingly, an important and perhaps less clearly articulated part of this model is that change requires the support of helping relationships. This can be the therapist and returns us to the importance of the therapeutic relationship. It also alerts us to the importance of thinking about therapy in systemic terms, for example, in recognizing that the converse of a supportive relationship is where people are in destructive and unhelpful relationships which can be extremely counterproductive to change. In systemic family therapy it is recognized that for change to occur it is not just the client but members of his or her family who need to be positively engaged with the therapy and have a reasonably positive working relationship with the therapist.

## CHAPTER SUMMARY

This chapter gives an overview of some of the major approaches to psychotherapy process research and the ways in which they can be used to explore our own and others' practice. Some of these studies are small scale and others clearly require substantial research resources. However, we feel that the care concepts can be adapted to inspire do-able, small scale studies of relevance to clinicians. As indicated at the start of the chapter there can be a danger in fragmenting the process when we attempt to isolate specific factors. Perhaps one of the key findings to emerge is that essentially therapy is a relationship, so our methods of enquiry need to be attuned to the study of interpersonal processes (see also Chapters 5, 7, 8 and 9). The study by Hilliard *et al.* (2000) emphasizes that possibly the therapeutic alliance stands out so clearly not simply because therapy is 'just' a good relationship but also because it represents a different kind of relationship to the dominant ones that people have 'introjected' and how they have come to treat themselves and others.

An important question for psychotherapy research is how to capture the richness of the process of therapy whilst at the same time being able to identify features that facilitate the process of change. Our examples have ranged over a variety of methods and also philosophies of research. For example, Rennie's work is one of the few examples of a collaborative approach. We want to argue that more such studies are required. In addition, there is a dearth of studies where clients are involved in the planning and analysis of data from studies. In our view, this is where we can all make a big difference, and in the context of small-scale enquiry. In the qualitative studies in this chapter by Rennie, Frosh *et al.* and Stith *et al.*, there are no indications of what the participants' views are, regarding the findings. The studies of significant events employ, like Rennie's studies, a collaborative form of exploration of sessions but still the final loop of feedback from our participants appears to be missing. We wonder whether this full inclusion of participants in the research process is a direction that will emerge in future psychotherapy process research. We hope so.

## KEY REFERENCES

Bergin, A. (2003) *Bergin and Garfield's Handbook of Psychotherapy and Behaviour Change*, 4th edn. New York: Wiley.

Coulehan, R., Friedlander, M. L. and Heatherington, L. (1988) Transforming narratives: a change event in constructivist family therapy, *Family Process*, 37: 17–33.

Davey, G. (2003) What is interesting isn't always useful, *Psychologist*, 16(8): 412–16.

Horvath, A. and Symonds, B. (1991) Relations between working alliance and outcome in psychotherapy, *Journal of Counselling Psychology*, 38: 139–49.

Llewelyn, S. P., Elliot, R., Shapiro, D. A., Hardy, G. and Firth-Cozens, J. (1988) Client perceptions of significant events in prescriptive and exploratory periods of individual therapy, *British Journal of Clinical Psychology*, 27: 105–14.

Winter, D. (2003) Repertory Grid Technique as a psychotherapy research measure, *Psychotherapy Research*, 13(1): 25–42.

# 7    SINGLE CASE AND CASE STUDY

# APPROACHES

## CHAPTER OVERVIEW

This chapter starts with an acknowledgement of the important contribution that case study research has made to the development of psychotherapy. We suggest that the case study is potentially one of the most 'do-able' of the various psychotherapy research frameworks available to clinicians since it shares many characteristics of a 'good clinical case study report'. Following a discussion of the core characteristics of case study research, an overview is offered of the major strands of research available, with detailed illustrations of these varieties. Connecting with the core themes of the book, readers are encouraged to consider these various methods in terms of the extent to which they facilitate and can be adapted to produce research that explores meaning and experience and is reflective, collaborative and do-able.

# INTRODUCTION

The development of psychotherapy owes a great deal to the case study. It is through case study evidence (see Chapter 5 on evaluation and outcome studies) that we have been able to look into the world of therapy and gain inspiration and evidence about different ways of treating problems. The descriptions of some clinical case studies, such as Freud's 'Wolf Man', 'Dora' or 'Anna O', have become an important part of modern-day culture (Freud, 1981). But case studies go back further than Freud. Prior to his work, there had also been descriptive accounts of the use of hypnosis in the work of Charcot and Breuer in the treatment of 'hysterical' illnesses (Wollheim, 1971). Case studies have also been employed extensively in neuro-psychological research. For example, in Oliver Sacks' (1985) memorable book *The Man Who Mistook His Wife for a Hat*, he offers powerful evocative examples of the experiences of people with severe neurological disorders, such as their perceptual aberrations and loss of memory. His vivid case study accounts caught the popular imagination in the manner in which they gave an insight into what it must be like to live with such conditions. Perhaps more than any other form of research, this insight into other people's worlds contains the power of case study research.

Case study research is defined as an investigation of a phenomenon in its real life context and complexity, that accepts there may be many variables involved and incorporates a range of sources of data. Yin (1994) makes the important point that case studies need not only be descriptive but can also be explanatory. By carefully following through in detail the complexity of a situation and the unfolding of events, it is possible to emerge with a strong causal explanation. As an illustration he cites Allison's research on the Cuban missile crisis, which weighed up the pros and cons of a number of competing theories about the crisis in the light of all the evidence available.

Though often fascinating, case study research has tended to be written from the perspective of the therapist. In some cases this has been illustrated by quotes or passages of conversation from the therapy. In particular, systemic family therapy pioneered the use of extracts of conversations between therapists and families to illustrate the nature of the therapeutic process (see, for example, Sluzki and Ransom, 1976). Yet these were accounts from the 'outside', and we want to encourage collaborative case study research that incorporates the perspectives of clients, family members and other people involved in the process of therapy. In addition, much case study research has either ignored or, at best, simply made assumptions about the experiences of clients. We want to encourage research that emphasizes experience and the co-creation of meaning in the therapeutic process. Furthermore, case study research, perhaps more than other forms of psychotherapy research, allows a consideration of the client's experience in the wider contexts of their relationships, community and cultural location. This allows a broader consideration of issues of power and inequality and whether the research process itself can be emancipatory in allowing, for example, an appraisal of the therapeutic services they receive, the assumptions that are made about them and even whether therapy can contribute to an increase, rather than a decrease, in their marginalization and disempowerment.

As in previous chapters, we offer an overview of methods of case study research but invite you to consider how these issues can be incorporated. As an example, even the relatively 'expert' and behaviourally oriented 'experimental' case study designs can be employed to explore the meaning of the treatment to clients in ways that incorporate an analysis of the meaning and experience of the therapy and how the approach can be used to empower clients by helping them gain insights into what particular aspects of the treatment have been helpful. This can empower them to utilize this understanding in dealing with future problems.

## RESEARCH OR CLINICAL REPORTS?

Case study research offers one of the most do-able forms of research for busy clinicians. Part of the reason for this is that the line between research and clinical case reporting can be a fine one. Arguably, whenever we present a clinical case study in detail and with substantial evidence of the work involved it constitutes a piece of research – though many clinicians do not realize they have been doing research for years! Good case study reports can be seen to make an important addition to the accumulation of evidence about particular therapies in various contexts. Perhaps one key difference is that many clinicians do not publish their case study reports or that the pressures of time constrain them to only being able to write brief summaries of their clinical work.

To be more specific we can draw out some necessary criteria for a 'case report' to count as a research case study:

1 Detailed and systematic exploration of one or more therapeutic cases.
2 Clear and detailed description of the context and the range of variables involved in the therapeutic situation. This would involve details of the setting, local and social context, reasons for the referral and referral pathways, background to the problems, client's background, therapeutic agency context and so on.
3 Theoretical framework guiding the research that can be explored, tested or elaborated by evidence from the case study.
4 Triangulation – multiple perspectives and multiple methods employed, for example, therapist's accounts, client's verbatim accounts, standardized measures, accounts from other professionals and family members, observations from a number of sources and so on.
5 Validity – measures taken to support the validity of the evidence presented, such as evidence of self-reflection, corroboration of evidence, independent analysis of the evidence, use of participant's reflections, member validation and so on.
6 Alternative explanations of the evidence considered and appraised.
7 Presentation of supporting evidence in the form of transcripts, data from participants and detailed observations.

8 Longitudinal analysis – case considered over a period of time, allowing repeated observations.

This is not a comprehensive list but includes some of the major criteria for a research case study. However, it could be argued that these are also requirements for a good case report. Criterion 1 is perhaps the most salient in offering a differentiation, in that it is the degree and complexity of the evidence that turns a case report into a research case study and protects it from the criticism of 'author claims' to the effectiveness of a new therapeutic method.

## TYPES OF CASE STUDY RESEARCH

Case studies can be employed in psychotherapy research to evaluate different theoretical perspectives. In particular, they can be very powerful in refuting theories. For example, failure of a therapeutic approach to achieve change in one representative case or an extreme case can result in the need to revise or at least adjust the therapeutic approach. The case study can also help to point to particular reasons why the therapy may have been ineffective. For example, Don Jackson described how his failure with a young woman who was anxious and depressed led him to consider relational factors. He discovered that when she improved her partner became depressed and his depression ameliorated as she again became depressed. This observation, based on a case, contributed to his development of the concept of family homeostasis. This was the view that relationships can be seen to develop a dynamic balance around a symptom so that change either way, for better or worse, appears to be resisted. The stuckness, therefore, is not simply *in* the person but is a part of an interpersonal process (Jackson, 1957).

This and other similar examples can be seen as practice based evidence drawn from case studies. Such evidence has an immediacy and an ability to connect with a clinician's own experiences. This perhaps makes it one of the most convincing forms of evidence for clinicians. In a biblical sense, it captures the 'miracle' of therapy in a way that statistics and randomized control trials cannot. Also, when case studies are presented in vivid detail they give the reader a picture and an idea of how to do it themselves and this sense of it being 'do-able' contributes to its potency as evidence.

This tradition continues with case studies often being employed to demonstrate new clinical approaches. For example, descriptive case studies have been employed to demonstrate client-centred therapy and CBT. Some approaches, notably systemic family therapy, have added to therapists' descriptions of treatment by providing verbatim transcripts of sessions. Later these came to be supported by video and audio-tapes of the sessions. More recent approaches, such as CAT and narrative therapies, have also provided detailed case study accounts of sessions. In addition to offering a demonstration of how a new approach works, such case studies offer a legitimate form of research data regarding the effectiveness of the sessions and also of the process of how the treatment may be working.

Significantly, case study research is also important because it offers a practicable and relatively inexpensive form of research. It offers a way of blending practice with research. Rather than embarking on a time-consuming research programme, case studies offer a way of carrying out research whilst conducting clinical work. They represent a practical version of the reflective scientist–practitioner model of clinical practice. Also, the underlying philosophy of case studies fits with clinical approaches which emphasize individual uniqueness and therapy as a complex interactional process.

Case studies can be viewed within idiographic research perspectives rather than nomothetic approaches which try to make broad generalizations about psychotherapy. However, case study approaches can complement nomothetic approaches. For example, a major trial of a psychotherapeutic approach can be informed by detailed analyses, and in particular analyses of exceptional cases, or where the therapy was ineffective or even counterproductive. Also, case studies can employ both qualitative and quantitative data. Case studies fall broadly into three categories:

- Narrative case studies – these offer descriptions, interviews or verbatim transcripts of the session.
- Experimental case studies – these employ systematic variation of one or more variables in the therapy to offer an analysis of how the therapy works.
- Mixed studies – these can employ a combination of qualitative data along with experimental manipulations and quantitative measures.

These categories can be broken down further, as summarized opposite.

## Narrative case studies

Narrative case studies embrace approaches which tell a story about the therapy. They usually aim to give a more holistic picture, which gives a sense of what happened and also some insight into what the experience was like. Arguably, they also offer a powerful addition to the question of replication. A rich description can be helpful to other clinicians in being able to do what is described. Sometimes some quite small visual details can mean the difference between an approach making or not making sense to the reader. Narrative case studies may differ along a dimension of how internal or external the accounts are to the client (see Fig. 7.1).

The case study can offer a description by the therapist of what they perceive to have taken place in therapy. Such accounts would constitute a relatively external account. If they are supported by various forms of data – for example by quotes of verbatim sections of conversation that occurred in the therapy – they can be seen as further along the continuum in Fig. 7.1. At the internal end reflections by clients about their experiences of therapy can be seen.

| Narrative case studies | Offer a descriptive account of the therapy. They tell the story of what has taken place and can include a holistic picture of the client, therapist and their contexts. They can also include multiple accounts: therapist, client, friends, family and other professionals involved. |
|---|---|
| Experimental case studies | These systematically alter factors involved in therapy so that the therapeutic process in itself becomes a form of experimental research. The research can be on an individual piece of therapy or multiple cases. |
| Diary studies | These involve clients and therapists keeping systematic records in the form of diaries of their experiences over a course of therapy. This allows a systematic recording of the therapy and a longitudinal picture of changes and experiences. |
| Personal construct case studies | These studies utilize George Kelly's personal construct theory to offer a detailed picture of the client's and therapist's constructs – beliefs and understandings, and how these change over the course of therapy. The focus is on the client's own personal system of meanings and the shifts that occur in these. |
| Personal questionnaires | In these studies questionnaires are developed in collaboration with clients which consist of items featuring the areas in which they wish to achieve change. The items can then be used quantitatively or qualitatively to chart progress of therapy and can be employed to compare client and therapist perceptions. |

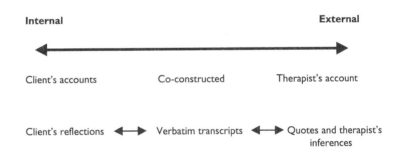

**Figure 7.1**  Narrative studies: internal versus external dimensions

## Clients' reflections

We will start with this because it has arguably been relatively marginal in the history of case study research. Traditionally, clients were often regarded as too 'ill' or 'confused' to have much to say about their experiences. Furthermore, within some therapies, such as traditional psychodynamic approaches, clients' accounts were not to be trusted since they were seen to be peppered with defensive processes and distortions. In effect, what they said needed to be made sense of by an 'expert' therapist.

One of the pioneers of an alternative approach which placed the client centre-stage is David Rennie (1992). The procedure in this form of research is that a client brings a recording of a previous therapy session (usually no more than one week previously) with them and listens to this with the researcher. The client takes the lead in commenting, reflecting on any aspect of this they think is important. At times the researcher may invite the client to comment on a section that he or she has found to be of interest. The interview lasts between two and four hours and can produce up to 40–80 pages of transcript. Rennie employed a grounded theory analysis to construct themes from these accounts. Based on an initial multiple case study employing 14 people, he concluded that four major themes could be identified:

- Client's relationship with personal meaning
- Client's perception of the relationship with the therapist
- Client's experience of the therapist's operations
- Client's experience of outcomes.

The findings of his study are outlined in Research Example 7.1.

---

**Research Example 7.1**

Rennie, D. L. (1992) Qualitative analysis of client's experience of the psychotherapy: the unfolding of reflexivity, in S. G. Toukmanins and D. Rennie (eds) *Psychotherapy Process Research: Paradigmatic and Narrative Approaches*. London: Sage.

An overarching theme of the study was noted to be reflexivity. This was defined as the client's ability to 'turn back in the self'. It included the idea that clients were actively thinking about what happens in therapy, that they had self-awareness and ideas about what they needed and what was right for them and that they weighed up what they should do in the therapy situation, including whether they should comment on aspects of what was going on and whether they should do what was suggested and what was right for them. Also, the accounts indicated that the clients held ideas about the therapist's intentions, how the therapist saw them, how the therapist thought they saw them and about how and why their perceptions and feelings about the therapist may have shifted. An example of a part of a transcript is reproduced below:

> I know that I hate this part. . . . When we started doing the two chairs, and I start acting out what I'm feeling and getting into emotions. I can't stand it. But I don't normally resist. A couple of times I will say, and I will stop it. But normally I hate it and he knows I hate it and I tell him I hate it but I do it anyway. I'm not really resisting. So that's what we're doing. It's just a bit of a joke that I really hate it.
> (Rennie, 1992, p. 223)

The account was from a professional woman in her mid-thirties. She also commented that although she had this negative reaction this was at only one level of experience. At another she realized that it was important for her to get into her feelings. Hence her resistance was really a game because she had decided that she should not in fact resist.

Rennie comments that clients are continually making such reflective decisions about whether and how much to tell, comment on or disagree with in the course of therapy. He also points out that clients and therapists frequently misunderstand each other and are on different wavelengths: 'Unless research strategies are used that access this reflexivity, the researcher's understandings of clients' processing will be either incomplete or misguided' (Rennie, 1992, p. 227).

Such case studies acknowledge that clients are capable of complex reflective processes and, importantly that they reflect on what the therapist is doing and why. They may at times recognize disjunctions where they partly disagree with what the therapist is suggesting but decide it is in their best interests to agree. However, at other times they may be less sure that it is of any real benefit to them and come to distrust the therapist but do not express these thoughts. Rennie suggests that such research argues against the notion of clients as having lost their sense of agency and instead recognizes that though potentially fragile it remains and is central to their progress: 'The challenge of therapy is to control sensitively what clients cannot control and to work productively with the ways in which they assume control' (Rennie, 1992, p. 231).

## Therapists' reflections supported by extracts from sessions

Rennie's work specifically asks clients to reflect on the process and experience of therapy. In effect, they can be seen as co-researchers. A more typical use of narrative case study is to employ extracts from sessions to illuminate concepts and indicate the nature of the therapeutic process. An example is given in Research Example 7.2 from a piece of systemic therapy which integrates ideas for attachment and narrative therapies. The use of verbatim extracts allows an illustration of the application of concepts in the practice of therapy. The intention is to assist the reader to gain an insight into what happens in the process of therapy. Specifically, this is facilitated by giving a picture of the interactional sequences and conversational processes, as well as an outline of the content or semantic features of the therapy. Typically, clients have not been included in the analysis of such extracts, though this is potentially very valuable as we saw in Chapter 6. Many of the therapies have offered case studies with extracts from sessions to illustrate an approach or to illuminate particular features. This can be achieved by keeping detailed notes of sessions and/or using audio or video recordings.

### Research Example 7.2

Frosh, S., Burck, C., Strickland-Clark, L. and Morgan, K. (1996) Engaging with change: a process study of family therapy, *Journal of Family Therapy*, 18: 141–61.

The research was part of a project to explore the work of experienced family therapists who knew that their work could be used for such research. The aim was to explore ' knowledge in use' in therapy and look at what happens in sessions rather than relying on therapists' accounts.

The study involved an exploration of family therapy with a family attempting to deal with the process of separation. The referral was initiated by the mother after the father had left the family and she was concerned about the negative effects on the children. The father agreed to attend, albeit 'reluctantly' at first. It appeared that he had made the decision to leave and any discussion of this and the impact on the family was regarded by him as possibly challenging his decision. His wife felt there were many issues that needed to be sorted out and talked about – that the change needed to be 'managed' and made sense of – whereas her husband felt that changes would follow naturally as a consequence of the change in their relationship.

As is standard practice in family therapy, all the sessions were recorded and six were transcribed for detailed analysis. A form of grounded theory analysis was employed to draw out dominant themes in the family's conversations with the therapist and each other. This resulted in two major themes: 'engagement with therapy' and 'attitude to change'. The theme 'attitude to change' was chosen as the focus and, in addition, there was an attempt to draw out how this was enacted in sessions and how it developed over the sessions. Through the use of an examination of the main themes and how these are played out in the details of their conversations, the researchers attempted to map the process of change over the course of the sessions.

Detailed extracts were employed to illustrate the process of change: Mother – Lucy, Father – Martin, Children – Ben (12) and Angela (14)

*Session 1:*

| | |
|---|---|
| *Therapist*: [to Lucy] | OK – fine and you initiated the coming here, is that right? |
| *Lucy*: | Yes. |
| *Therapist*: [to Martin] | Was that after a discussion with you, as well? |
| *Martin*: | Not this appointment. |
| *Therapist*: [to Martin] | So, when did you know about coming along? |
| *Martin*: | . . . When Lucy showed me a letter, two – a couple of weeks ago. |
| *Therapist*: | So, was that OK for you? |
| *Martin*: | I'm slightly . . . Unwilling. |

The idea that change had happened too fast and needed to be managed was seen to be a strategic struggle between the couple. The husband perhaps wanted to be out of the marriage, while his wife was still hoping for some possible reconciliation, and she was arguing for a more realistic stance that incorporated the needs not just of them as a couple but also of the children:

| | |
|---|---|
| *Lucy*: | Well, my . . . view is that . . . this whole . . . sort of . . . separation issue and the relationship break-up has actually come – according . . . er – very fast and . . . I mean . . . and I think the reason I wanted this session was . . . to make sure that Angela and Ben were not . . . well, sort of had the situation somewhat sorted out in their minds . . . |

| | |
|---|---|
| *Martin:* | . . . I um – I . . . I don't feel that I have anything to hold on to as yet . . . as far as a . . . need for coming here . . . it's as if we might be provoking things to hold onto instead of . . . [tailing off] . . . seeing what they are first . . . |

The children also indicate that they see things according to this shared perception of their parents – of their father as 'waiting to see what happens':

| | |
|---|---|
| *Ben:* | Well, I understand . . . my dad hasn't been very good at developing relationships with other people, but that's usually because people have developed relationships with him, rather than him developing relationships with other people. |

The therapist is also seen as commenting on her relationship with the family members as a vehicle for commenting on their roles and similarities, for example that Ben is also reluctant to initiate relationships and conversations, like his father:

*Session 2:*

| | |
|---|---|
| *Ben:* | I didn't even speak much so . . . [tails off – inaudible] |
| *Therapist:* [laughing] | Is that your safety position, Ben, when you are not sure – I mean it sounds to me like you're . . . [Martin tries to say something] like you feel OK to talk today, is that right? |
| *Ben:* | It's just the same as last time: if I'm asked a question I'll answer it, really. |
| *Martin:* | It's the art of . . . |
| Therapist: | God, you're just like your dad . . .! |
| *Martin:* | It's the art of . . . |
| *Therapist:* | You make me work really hard! |
| *Martin:* | . . . art of the refined shrug. That's why I'm a good teacher, you see: I make everyone else work for it. |

Extracts are employed with commentary to track the process of change in the family. In the final session the authors note that it appeared that their positions of how change happens had altered to a position where Lucy (mother) was not the only one who predominantly thought that change could be planned and managed:

| | |
|---|---|
| *Therapist:* | Yeah. But in addition I wondered what you felt had come out of the . . . |
| *Lucy:* | It certainly helped get through it. |
| *Therapist:* | Angela? |
| *Angela:* | I think we can probably talk more easily together – now. It's come from this . . . which I think is good. |
| *Therapist:* | Is there anything that you would have liked to have done a bit differently? |

| *Angela*: | No. I think, you know, you can't really say what you want out of it, because it's . . . it comes along. |
| *Therapist*: | Ben? |
| *Ben*: | Fine. Works out. |

*Summary*: The analysis revealed how the therapist worked with the family to explore and elaborate a number of core themes, such as their views of change as needing to be 'managed' as opposed to something that occurs 'spontaneously'. The family members were organized around this theme in that the mother regarded the change of the father leaving the family as something that needed to be negotiated and discussed, whereas the father saw change as something that occurred through action and that making sense of it would follow later. The study offered extracts from the interviews which also revealed how the therapist employed comments on her own relationship with family members and humour to develop understandings relating to this core theme of 'managing change'.

One use of case study can be to illustrate descriptively a particular form of therapy. The case study attempts to offer adequate information to contextualize it in terms of its complexity and the variables that may be involved. In the example above it is possible to follow the authors' line of argument regarding how change has occurred in this particular case. The extracts are employed as evidence to support the analysis. However, they also provide material for the reader to contemplate whether alternative explanations are possible and give a more experiential insight into what this therapy felt like. This is especially highlighted by examples of the use of humour, which gives a flavour of the nature of the engagement with the family. In this case, in addition to the theory proposed about the management of change in the family, it could be suggested that the case study illustrated the importance of the therapeutic relationship in helping this family go through the painful experience of separation.

The case study is also located within a theoretical framework. It is employed to illustrate and support a particular theoretical orientation or some aspect of a therapeutic approach. Research Example 7.3 is an example of employing a case study to illustrate what a variety of therapy (systemic therapy integrated with ideas from attachment and narrative therapy) looks like in practice. In addition, the case study is used to support the proposition that this is an effective approach with a particular variety of problems. Many of the therapies have used case studies in such ways. Perhaps family therapy has been one of the pioneers in offering detailed extracts from sessions since it was the first of the therapies to employ recording of sessions as standard clinical practice. The piece is taken from part of the case study which illustrates the four-stage approach to therapy with families, with an example of a treatment of a young woman and her family suffering with an eating disorder.

**Research Example 7.3**

Dallos, R. (2004) Attachment narrative therapy: integrating ideas from narrative and attachment theory in systemic family therapy with eating disorders, *Journal of Family Therapy*, 26(1): 40–66.

Mary, aged 19, was attending an eating disorder unit as a day patient following a three-month period as an in-patient. She was living at home with her father (Bill) and older brother Peter who was drinking quite heavily, which was of some concern, especially to his mother. Mrs Morrison (June) was living with her mother and father nearby, having 'moved out' approximately six months before the start of Mary's anorexia. Mary had gone to university some distance away from the family home about four months after her mother had moved out. She quickly lost weight and had to return home after six weeks and was admitted to a local eating disorder unit.

*Creating a secure base:*
In the first phase of the therapy a non-blaming framework was offered, including an externalizing framework as to how we could all work together to resist the anorexia (see also Byng-Hall, 1995). It was made clear that the purpose of the sessions was not to look for blame and that we might never fully discover the causes. However, we would try to find ways of resisting the problem. The family were also asked how they felt about an approach where we did not spend all of the time in the sessions looking at the anorexia but also spent time on other matters:

| | |
|---|---|
| *Therapist:* | You have probably spent quite a bit of time trying to understand how the eating problems have come about. One of the things we find often is that the anorexia can start to eat away (looking to Mary) at the young person's life until there is hardly anything left. So, if it's OK with you maybe we could spend some of the time talking about the anorexia and some time talking about other things, friends, work, education – the future – so that when eventually we do manage to help Mary defeat the anorexia she will have a life ahead of her. In fact anorexia is more likely to linger or try to come back into your lives if a person is bored, lonely, frustrated or dissatisfied with the rest of their life. How does that sound to you all? |
| *Mary:* | [nodding in agreement] Yes, that sounds reasonable to me. |
| *Mr M:* | Whatever you think will help. |
| *Mrs M:* | Yes, she does want to do things. . . . |
| *Therapist:* | I am not talking about these things changing quickly . . . anorexia is very persistent and will keep trying to come back into Mary's life. It's a little bit |

|                | like a spiral you feel like you are going round in circles but at each turn you are going forward a little bit as well. Anorexia likes to divide families and we find that working together, offering a united front, can be helpful in keeping it at bay. It might be a tough, long struggle. . . . |
| Mr M:          | We will do whatever you think is helpful. . . . |

Such case studies attempt to convey the process of the therapy, along with the use of such extracts to offer validation of the suggested effectiveness of the approach. Furthermore, they allow the reader to gain an understanding of what the therapist did and said which they can employ to judge the validity of the author's conclusions. For example, whether the conclusions and the examples are consistent and coherent or whether it is possible to derive very different conclusions from the extracts offered.

Another frequent use of case studies is to provide evidence of the application of particular features or techniques in therapy (see Research Example 7.4).

---

**Research Example 7.4**

Salkovskis, P. (1989) Obsessions and compulsions, in J. Scott, J. M. G. Williams and A. T. Beck (eds) *Cognitive Therapy in Clinical Practice*. London: Routledge.

Mr Johnstone was an obsessional patient who was troubled by the thought that he had offered activities to the devil. He described aspects of his strict Roman Catholic upbringing . . . as a child he was extensively warned about the dangers of impure thoughts. During his late teens he rebelled against these ideas and behaved very much as he wanted. He was troubled by a great deal of guilt and, as he settled down, he began to believe that he had offered his 'wild living' to the devil. As this thought grew, he began to have another thought – that he would offer everyday activities to the devil. . . . He tried to neutralize these thoughts by . . . saying prayers in ritualized ways. . . .

*Therapy session 10:*

| *Therapist:*    | You have doubts as to whether the thoughts are true or whether they are obsessions. |
| *Mr Johnstone:* | The main problem I had with previous treatments was that I was given techniques to change the direction of my thoughts when I was ritualizing and I thought I could kill my conscience by learning a trick. I worry about the harm that I had done by offering things to the devil or thought I had offered things to the devil and not put right; I would have to put them right when I thought that way. |

|  | Rationalizing things are just obsessions that could kill my conscience. Where things to me are real, I can't think of them as irrational. |
| *Therapist*: | And therefore— |
| *Mr Johnstone*: | Then I haven't the confidence to stop putting right, you've got to do the absolution. |
| *Therapist*: | If you do kill your conscience then what? |
| *Mr Johnstone*: | Then I will be living an anti-religious life, I would really be offering things to the devil because I haven't neutralized it. |
| *Therapist*: | So that leaves us two possibilities. Either the thoughts are correct and you could be living the life of an anti-Christ; or that you have an obsessional problem. Are these the two possibilities you see, and swing between them? |
| *Therapist*: | Let's write these down [writes]: first, 'my problem is obsessions'; second, 'my problem is sin, calling this obsessions is killing my conscience'. Look at these, do you agree these are the possibilities? |
| *Mr Johnstone*: | Totally. |
| *Therapist*: | Right, now look at the first one; could you rate how likely that is to be true, using 0 to 100, where 0 is no truth at all, 100 is completely true. |
| *Mr Johnstone*: | Well, the first one about 30 per cent now; when they happen, only 10 per cent. The second one, 70 per cent now, nearly 100 per cent when they happen. |
| *Therapist*: | OK, so you are not completely sure either way, although this can vary. Could both be true? |
| *Mr Johnstone*: | Definitely not. Only one of these can be correct. |

In considering these extracts we are including a broader conception of case study research. This fits the notion of 'practice based evidence' and such material in the form of extracts can be seen as research material. However, arguably, the more it is presented predominantly to support the therapist's interpretation without taking into account possible alternative explanations, or uses little in the way of quotes or contextual material, the more it loses its power as research. However, it may also lose its legitimacy as a case report!

## Experimental single-case studies

Arguably, these types of research case studies have their origins in behavioural research, especially studies of operant conditioning (Skinner, 1953). Such studies explored how individual organisms learnt under various conditions and, in particular how they responded to various schedules of rewards or punishments. Each organism acted in effect as their own control so that the process of learning could be identified in detail. Skinner's research, for example, involved detailed visual representations in the form of graphs of how learning occurred. This procedure has now become common parlance in the expression 'learning curves'. As a classic example, it was found that intermittent or unpredictable patterns of rewards produced learning or conditioning that was very resistant to extinction once the rewards were removed. Nomothetic generalizations become possible as evidence accumulated from individual cases. Hence the experimental case designs can offer both idiographic data about the process of therapy and evaluative data in terms of its effectiveness.

The designs require that we start with a formulation of the problems in terms of what particular factors are maintaining the problems. Subsequently, there is a clear specification as to how particular interventions will alter these factors and produce changes. Essential to the research is a thorough analysis of the current nature of the difficulties in terms of severity, frequency and variation. This requires that a 'baseline' is established in relation to these factors over a substantial period of time. For example, if it is reported that the problems fluctuate daily but also show cyclical changes every week then the baseline needs to be long enough – for example, six weeks – to offer a picture of these variations (Barlow and Hersen, 1984; Morley and Adams, 1989).

A variety of designs are employed, as detailed below.

## AB Design

This is the most basic design and consists of recording a baseline for a period of time followed by an intervention period. As an example, parents who ask for advice on how to manage their eight-year-old son who is having angry outbursts may be asked to record how frequently the outbursts happen. Following this they are encouraged to try a new way of responding, such as ignoring the negative behaviours but providing rewards when the boy behaves appropriately. The frequencies of the behaviours are mapped on a chart and, when effective, this is typically very obvious (see Fig 7.2).

## ABAB or reversal designs

Though helpful the simple AB design is not convincing in terms of causal explanations. Even though it may be likely that the intervention did cause the effect, it is possible that some other factor may have come into play. For example, it is possible that the boy is behaving better because a family relative has come to stay, because he is looking forward to a school trip or even because he is physically ill and too tired to engage in the disruptive behaviours. The reversal design attempts to deal with this issue by reversing the intervention in terms of inserting a period of return to no treatment. If the behaviour increases but then reduces again following the intervention, this lends convincing evidence that the intervention is causing the change (see Fig. 7.3).

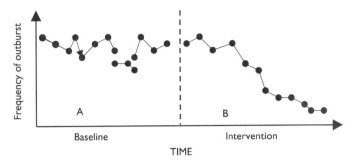

**Figure 7.2**   Example of an AB design

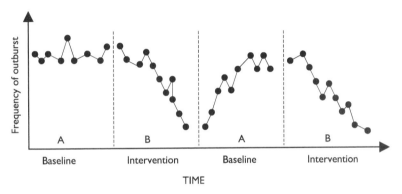

**Figure 7.3**   Example of a reversal design

Though expedient in terms of providing evidence of causal factors involved in change, there are serious problems in using such designs in clinical research. The assumptions that the behaviours are reversible may only apply in specific cases where they are very much maintained by environmental variables. However, where the therapy involves insight or changes in understanding, these would not be expected simply to reverse. Very importantly, the design can also be unethical in that it would be inappropriate to cease treatment if this is likely to lead to the person once again being distressed and troubled.

*Multiple baseline designs*

In many clinical situations the client, couple or family are suffering with a range of problems and/or their problems may vary across different situations. For example, a child may behave differently at home, in the classroom, in the playground, with relatives and so on. One way of exploring these variables across problems or settings is to design interventions which are specifically targeted at each of them and are introduced in turn. Baseline recordings are derived for each of the variables or situations and, subsequently, each intervention is introduced one at a time. The timing of

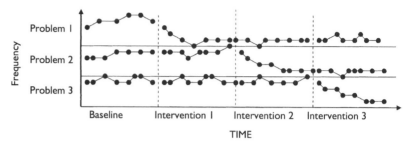

**Figure 7.4**    Example of a multiple baseline design

the intervention should coincide with change in the variable it is intended to target but not in the others (see Fig. 7.4).

In Fig. 7.4 we can see that as each intervention is introduced in turn, the target problem reduces. Of course, this is a hypothetical example and it is rare that the effects are so clear. In many cases the effects of various interventions have a more general or subtle impact. Statistical techniques are available for the analysis of such designs (Barlow and Hersen, 1984; Morley and Adams, 1989).

A study of narrative therapy shows how, with imagination, such designs can be applied to therapies that are a long way removed from the behavioural principles on which these experimental designs were initially introduced (see Research Example 7.5).

There are a number of other single case experimental designs, for example the changing criterion design. These are particularly appropriate where change is likely to be a gradual process and may need to occur in stages. For example, in alcohol addiction programmes the first intervention may be to reduce the drinking to a less medically dangerous level. Subsequent therapeutic inputs may be targeted at helping to shift thinking and per-ceived need for drinking, or may focus on the marital relationship as a way of producing the next phase of diminution in drinking.

## Diary studies

The use of diaries can be a component of n=1 experimental case study designs or a component of narrative case studies (Bolger *et al.*, 2003). For example, in the former, clients may be asked to keep a diary of certain aspects of their problems. One approach is to ask clients to record the subjective units of distress (SUDs) on a daily basis. This involves an initial discussion of what the difficulties are and what experiences are involved and working with the client to be able to clarify and subjectively quantify their differing levels of distress. This helps to ensure that there is a con-sistency and reliability within their subjective experience. Such diary keeping is, of course, a central feature of CBT approaches. Here they have the double purpose of generating data for research and helping clients develop different ways of thinking about their problems. In CBT research the diary keeping involves recording incidents in terms of counting or frequency of

## Research Example 7.5

Bem, D. (1994) Evaluating narrative family therapy: using single-system research designs, *Research on Social Work Practice*, 4(3): 309–25.

Figure 7.5 represents an exploration of narrative family therapy with 'Jack' and his family. Two behaviours were chosen by the family as targets for interventions: phone calls made to his mother at work; and the amount of screaming that resulted from his younger brother as a result of his teasing and hitting him. Jack had been diagnosed as having ADHD. One of his 'hyperactive' behaviours was phone calls to his mother at work, which could occur up to six times a day, and the family wanted to target this to help reduce the escalating phone bills.

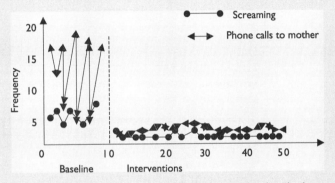

**Figure 7.5**   Using multiple baseline design in narrative family therapy

The therapy consisted of a number of narrative techniques, including externalizing, relative influence questions and problem definitions. However, the emphasis was specifically on the use of 'unique outcomes', whereby the therapist focuses on successes that have been achieved, exceptions to the problems, new (unique) descriptions of the child and problems, and future possibilities. In some aspects this might be seen to resemble behavioural interventions which emphasize reinforcing positive behaviours. However, in narrative therapy this technique is seen as helping to build new, less 'problem saturated' descriptions. The introduction of the unique outcomes aspect of narrative therapy appears to have clearly been associated with change in the key problems that family members had identified.

This study consisting of a study of six families, all of whom showed significant changes as charted in this manner.

events along with a recording of thoughts and feelings and their assessment on a scale, for example, 0 to 100 per cent (see Table 7.1).

Such diary keeping can, therefore, offer quantitative indications of changes which can be analysed using single-case study statistical methods (Morley and Adams, 1989).

**Table 7.1**   Example of the use of a diary in CBT

| Situation | Emotion | Automatic thoughts | Rational response | Outcome |
|---|---|---|---|---|
| Woke up thinking of how I usually enjoyed all the Christmas preparations and music, and how near Christmas is | Flat low (100%) | I won't be able to cope with Christmas preparation (90%) | I managed to write a letter last week. I have about 100 cards to write. I'll ring my father and ask him to bring some cards and we could start on that tonight. I'll see how I get on. It's better to withhold judgement about whether I can cope or whether I'll enjoy myself until I try (50%) | Hopeful (20%) Low (30%) |

From Blackburn, I. M. (1989).

Diary studies can be employed in a more detailed and qualitative way by asking clients to keep detailed accounts of their thoughts, feelings and actions during the course of therapy. This can offer a picture not just of the more immediate impact of the therapy but also of how it impacts on the client's life and how life events impact on or interact with the effects of the therapy. Interestingly, such diary keeping has frequently been found to have a beneficial effect in itself (Barker *et al.*, 2002). In strategic family therapy diary keeping involving detailed observation of the symptom, and its variation according to various family events, came to be employed as a 'paradoxical' intervention (Haley, 1987). The task of observation was regarded as interfering with the ability to engage in the symptomatic behaviour.

Research Example 7.6 outlines a journal study charting the experience of psychotherapy.

**Research Example 7.6**

Woskett, K. (1999) *The Therapeutic Use of Self*. Hove: Brunner-Routledge.

The study involved the counsellor (Val) and client (Rachel) keeping a separate record of their sessions over a period of 18 months (47 sessions were recorded). The accounts were written independently within 48 hours of each session. The counsellor had worked with the client previously and knew she liked writing and was good at this activity. The client was in her late 50s and had experienced severe mental health problems previously, depression, alcoholism and had been a psychiatric in-patient and had been administered ECT. One of her acute periods of distress followed the ending of a significant lesbian relationship.

Care was taken over ethical issues, such as confidentiality, informed consent and power issues in the request for participation, especially that not agreeing to participate would not in any way jeopardize her therapy.

Writing of the accounts was prompted by a number of story stem prompts:

| | |
|---|---|
| *Client:* | The most significant thing about the session for me was. . . . |
| *Counsellor:* | The most significant thing about the session for me was. . . . |
| *Client:* | Something I found helpful was. . . . |
| *Counsellor:* | Something I think my client found helpful was. . . . |

The accounts were not examined until the therapy had finished, at the client's request after 47 sessions. It was felt that to share the accounts during the counselling might have imposed an additional burden for Rachel of taking into account her counsellor's feelings when she needed to focus on and be supported with her own feelings.

The analysis consisted of a form of theme analysis, in which dominant themes from both sets of accounts were generated. Along with this there was a focus on similarities and differences in the perceptions of what had happened and been more or less useful in the sessions. Three major themes were identified: love, touch and sexuality; errors, mistakes and omissions made by the counsellor; and extra-therapeutic factors occurring at the boundaries of the counselling work.

Examples of the first theme and some of the different experiences are illustrated with quotes, for example:

| | |
|---|---|
| *Val:* | My sense is that I will need to be very tolerant and secure in the face of what might be Rachel's desperate need for a good mother. |
| *Rachel:* | My felt need for physical comfort with another human being is a constant aching void and because it feels so huge I don't feel able to ask for it and I think when I'm in a relationship this need for physical comfort gets confused with sexual desire. |

Many of the comparisons of the accounts within the themes indicated aspects of what is 'unsaid' in counselling as well as how the client and counsellor's reflections showed a realization of schisms and ruptures. The therapist here observed that Rachel may have experienced her as detached and professional, but in fact she was experiencing despondency and was distressed in the face of Rachel's enormous despair.

## Personal construct theory case studies

Personal construct theory (PCT) emphasizes that each person is actively involved in making choices in their lives based on their personal system of beliefs or construct system (Kelly, 1955). Arguably, PCT is one of the most systematic and radical of the idiographic approaches. Both as a research tool and as a therapeutic approach PCT adopts a case study approach. Its approach fundamentally suggests that our understanding of therapeutic change must proceed on the basis of detailed explorations of changes in people's construct systems. There are many good summaries of PCT (Bannister and Fransella, 1971), but some of the key premises are:

- People are like 'scientists' in that each of us is actively engaged in forming hypotheses about our world in order to predict it and manage our lives.
- Our hypotheses are based on constructs which are bipolar dimensions of meanings, such as kind–cruel, calm–emotional, patient–hasty and so on.
- Our constructs are organized hierarchically but each of us has a unique system and organization of constructs.
- Constructs regarding the self are central in our system of beliefs.

Importantly, Kelly (1955) and later construct theorists have developed a number of ways of mapping people's construct systems. One of the most widely used techniques is the repertory grid. A detailed summary of the applications of PCT as a psychotherapy research tool is offered by Winter (2003). One of the most common approaches is to employ the *role construct repertory grid* – a grid with the person and key figures in their lives – a number of times during therapy to map change and progress. One aspect of this might be to focus on how the difference between self and ideal self, often widely differing at the start of therapy, becomes reconciled. Winter comments that a substantial number of studies have found significant changes in the reduction of the distance between the self and ideal self over the duration of therapy in a variety of forms of psychotherapy, including CBT, behaviour therapy, psychodynamic therapy, CAT (cognitive analytic therapy), personal construct psychotherapy and group therapy. Many studies also report changes such that clients come to see themselves as more like others, less odd, more identified with others – what Winter calls the 'welcome to the human race' effect.

However, the use of grids can provide a very rich yet systematic picture of how change occurs. One of the key techniques is the repertory grid which offers a matrix of the person's view of the world. There are numerous versions of grids but perhaps the most widely used is the role repertory grid which consists of people who play a key part in our lives as the *elements* and a set of *constructs* or beliefs derived from these elements. The constructs are elicited by inviting participants to think about these key people in their life three at a time and asked; 'how are two of these three people similar and different to the third?' how are two similar and the third different? This process serves to draw out distinctions and place these as bipolar constructs, such as friendly versus hostile, practical vs creative and so on. The constructs are then employed to score each element so that eventually there is a grid, usually 10 × 10 mapping the person's view about these important people in their life. Included in the elements are self and ideal self, and comparisons between these on the various constructs immediately provides a picture of what changes the person might desire. Similarities and differ-ences between these and other elements indicate perceived similarities and also interpersonal conflicts in the person's life. An example is given in Fig. 7.6.

We can see from Fig. 7.6 that the person has relatively close agreement between his rating on his ideal self and actual self, suggesting that he has a reasonable level of self-esteem. Agreement between other elements can also be seen, for example between self and his father. The aim of the grid is to 'get inside' our participant's mind, partly by employing his own language – his personal constructs. Importantly, the constructs are not logically pre-dictable; for example, the opposite of assertive is seen as weak rather than not assertive. Furthermore, repertory grids offer a picture of meanings in the context of the elements. In effect, this fits with Wittgenstein's dictum about 'letting the use of a word teach us its meaning'.

We can see what the different construct words mean for this person in the context of these important relationships in his life. In contrast, a question-naire or an interview would not allow us to see the subtlety of the con-nections between constructs and elements in this way. The grids can be analysed in various ways, including sophisticated factor analysis (see below). This can extract clusters of correlations between elements and

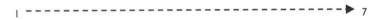

**ELEMENTS**

| CONSTRUCT | Self | Mother | Brother | Sister | Best friend | Boss | Father | Uncle | Girlfriend | Ideal self | CONSTRUCT |
|---|---|---|---|---|---|---|---|---|---|---|---|
| Happy | 4 | 5 | 7 | 5 | 2 | 4 | 3 | 3 | 4 | 2 | Unhappy |
| Trusting | 3 | 3 | 3 | 2 | 4 | 5 | 3 | 5 | 2 | 3 | Not trusting |
| Outgoing | 5 | 5 | 6 | 5 | 2 | 5 | 6 | 5 | 4 | 6 | Inward |
| Lazy | 6 | 6 | 5 | 5 | 6 | 6 | 6 | 5 | 5 | 6 | Works hard |
| Aggressive | 5 | 3 | 5 | 5 | 2 | 6 | 5 | 2 | 2 | 4 | Not aggressive |
| Assertive | 5 | 3 | 6 | 5 | 4 | 2 | 6 | 2 | 4 | 2 | Weak |
| etc. | | | | | | | | | | | |
| | | | | | | | | | | | |

**Figure 7.6**   Example of a repertory grid for psychotherapy process research

between constructs, and one analysis can plot these on the same semantic 'hyper-space' to give a visually accessible summary of the grid.

Repertory grids, therefore, offer a rich and personal account of a person's world and, importantly, how this may change during the process of therapy. One way of facilitating this view of change is to depict the grids on a two-dimension graph. Figure 7.7 illustrates changes in the construing of Gerry,

(a) Gerry: repertory grid prior to treatment

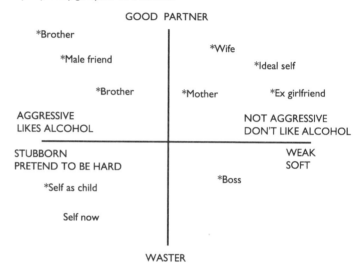

(b) Gerry: repertory grid post-treatment

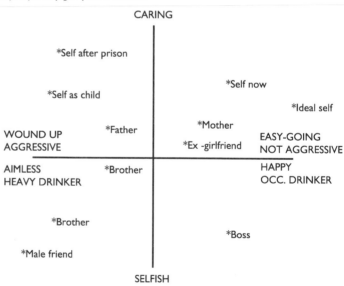

**Figure 7.7**  Graphical representation of changes in the construing of a client, Gerry, over the course of therapy
From Houston, J., 1998.

a man who had served a prison sentence for grievous bodily harm. He requested help to control his temper having previously had a long history of explosive violence, usually following heavy bouts of drinking. Typically, his initial construing reflected a stereotypical view of gender roles and of needing to be a 'real man' – tough, drinking and violent. His father encouraged these values and used to take his sons drinking down the pub with him from an early age. Initially his main way of construing people was whether they were aggressive, liked a drink and pretended to be hard.

It is possible changes in Gerry's grid maps post-treatment changes. For example, there is greater closeness between his self and ideal self and, importantly, he appeared to have been able to revise his beliefs about aggression and no longer saw being not aggressive as a sign of being weak and soft. He also appeared to see himself as more like the women than the men in his life. However, this could possibly contain some dilemmas for him since he may come to want male companionship. He may need to develop some new relationships with men who he can regard with respect, but who are not aggressive or heavy drinkers who may pull him back into his previously unhappy way of being in the world.

This offers a specific example of how PCT can be employed to map change in therapy. In this case, the therapy was influenced by PCT but the approach can be applied to explore the processes involved in a variety of psychotherapies.

Research Example 7.7 outlines a PCT analysis of CAT therapy for survivors of childhood sexual abuse.

---

**Research Example 7.7**

Clarke, C. and Llewelyn, S. (1994) Personal constructs of survivors of childhood sexual abuse receiving cognitive analytic therapy, *Journal of Medical Psychology*, 67: 273–89.

This study employed a personal construct theory framework using repertory grids to examine the effects of CAT for seven women who had experienced childhood sexual abuse. Five had experienced abuse by close family members and six had been re-abused by another person. A variety of standardized measures, including the BDI (Beck Depression Inventory, Beck *et al.*, 1979), SCL-90R (Derogatis *et al.* 1973), Rosenberg Self-Esteem Inventory (Rosenberg, 1965) and Jehu Belief Inventory (Jehu, 1988), were also employed.

The therapy was conducted by a female therapist trained in CAT and consisted of the standard 16 sessions (except for one client whose problems were less acute who received only eight sessions). The study was part of a broader attempt to examine what is helpful for survivors of sexual abuse. CAT specifically was chosen for a number of reasons: it is a collaborative approach involving a reformulation letter from the therapist to the client; the therapeutic relationship is employed as a vehicle to discuss problems in relationships; and patterns of thinking and feelings are traced back to early and ongoing relationships. The last of these, along with a discussion of the therapeutic relationship, is aimed towards assisting clients to avoid the risk of abusive relationships in the future.

Repertory grids were chosen in order to offer a detailed picture of possible changes in the women's views of themselves, the abuser and their relationships, importantly with the abuser and men in general. Two types of repertory grids were administered prior to and immediately following the therapy:

1  Single elements grids (role): self, ideal self, self as a child, childhood abuser, adult abuser, abuser, father, mother, partner, other men, other women (see Fig. 7.8).

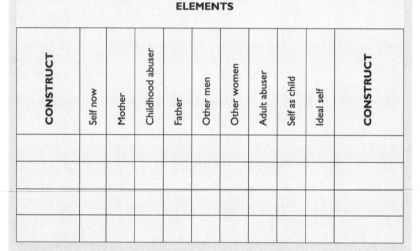

**Figure 7.8**  Single element grid

2  Dyad grids (these consist of relationships rather than single people as the elements): perceived relationship between themselves as a child and the first and second abuser, between adult self and the second abuser, adult self to men in general, child self to parents, relationships between mother and father (see Fig. 7.9).

Note that the dyads reverse so that each relationship has two parts, e.g. child's relationship with the childhood abuser and adult abuser's relationship with the child. The questions asked in elicitation of the grid are: 'As a child, how do you think you saw your relationship with the childhood abuser – someone you could trust? 'How do you think the childhood abuser saw their relationship with you – someone he could use and exploit?'

For both types of grids the elements were supplied, as were half of the constructs, based on an exploration of the clinical literature.

I  -------------------------------------- ▶  7

**ELEMENTS (RELATIONSHIPS)**

| CONSTRUCT | Child self and child abuser | Adult self and adult abuser | Adult self and men in general | Mother and father | Adult self and partner | Adult self and other women | Childhood abuser to child | Adult abuser to adult self | Men in general to adult self | etc. | CONSTRUCT |
|---|---|---|---|---|---|---|---|---|---|---|---|
| | | | | | | | | | | | |
| | | | | | | | | | | | |
| | | | | | | | | | | | |
| | | | | | | | | | | | |

**Figure 7.9**   Dyad grid

*Findings*: The authors concluded from the study that, although the standardized measures indicated that the women's levels of distress had decreased, the picture provided by the grid analyses was more complicated. Most broadly, the women construed the offenders as like their fathers, predictably since they had been abused by them or family members. However, they also saw abusers as like men in general. Though, on the one hand, this might appear positive, it can also be seen as leaving them vulnerable in terms of not expecting anything but abuse from any man and therefore, in a sense, not just expecting but also accepting this as inevitable. As an example, one of the women saw a close similarity between the constructs 'looks after' and 'used by'. In effect for her, there was still a confusion between a sense of being looked after and cared for and accepting that this would involve 'being used'. Another woman continued to regard 'assertive' as similar to 'abusive/horrible'. Such a construing possibly made it hard for her to accept the need to assert her own needs and wishes. Similarly, in terms of their perceptions of relationships, it was found that at the end of therapy four of the women still saw themselves as relating with men in general in a similar way to how they had related as a child to their childhood abuser. Three of the women also construed men in general as similar to how the abusers had related to them.

The authors suggest that this construing implies a restricted view of relationships with men still existed, which included an expectation and acceptance that male behaviour includes abuse. This could potentially render them vulnerable to further attacks. Furthermore, in relation to therapy, the authors pointed out that a construal of assertiveness in negative terms as 'horrible and abusive' would make the assertiveness programmes advocated in many treatments very difficult. They concluded: 'despite significant symptom reduction . . . The women appeared to remain locked into a limited view of relationships with men, in which they occupy a victim role' (Clarke and Llewelyn, 1994, p. 287).

Personal construct theory approaches offer an opportunity to explore the unique changes that occur in a process of psychotherapy. However, it is also possible to look at commonalities in the processes of change. For example, there are a number of general characteristics of construing which can be studied. We have seen that the distance between self and ideal self offers an important insight into how therapy changes some core aspects of self-regard. In addition to the content of the grids, it appears that some important structural changes are also evident. For example, as change occurs the grids appear to become more differentiated, so that the clustering is less narrow and rigid. Thus, Gerry's initial grid showed a tight grouping according to gender and this changes a little but still does reveal some polarization and rigidity. Such a grid can also be examined to show whether, as other studies suggest, successful therapy involves a move away from rigid, fixed thinking towards more flexible and adaptive thought processes. It is also possible to include the therapist in a grid, which can provide a useful picture of how the therapeutic relationship proceeds during therapy. Landfield (1971) employed a variety of construct measures to explore client and therapist construings of each other and found, for example, that some mutual similarity in their construing helped to establish a positive relationship. However, in addition to this, it was necessary that there was some meaningful difference in their construings and recognition of each other's construings as meaningful. In effect, this suggests that therapy requires a balance between being too far apart in how things are seen and a too cosy acceptance or agreement with each other's views.

Finally, it also possible to generalize across repertory grids if the same elements and constructs are given to people. This can allow generalizations, for example, that a particular client group, such as people with anorexia, typically regard themselves in a negative way and idealize their parents and have negative views about the value of talking about and expressing their feelings, and consequently negative expectations about therapy.

## Personal questionnaires

An approach which has some overlaps with construct theory is the use of a personal questionnaire to map progress in therapy. This shares with PCT the idea that it is important to examine therapy from the client's perspective and to employ dimensions which are meaningful to them rather than to try to impose these. The approach therefore starts with a discussion between the therapist and client(s) about what they regard as the key areas of difficulty or the problems which they want to work on. In effect, this amounts to a form of structured goal-setting of 'target problems'. These are then turned into statements rather like items in a standardized inventory, but now they have been derived from the clients themselves rather than imposed on them. Importantly, this forms a *shared* framework which both client and therapist can employ to compare their perceptions of the progress of therapy.

There are various procedures that can then be adopted to use and score the items. It is possible to use the dimensions to map progress from one session to the next, by administering the questionnaire at the end of each session and asking the client to rate how he/she feels on each dimension. (See Research Example 7.8.)

---

**Research Example 7.8**

Parry, G., Shapiro, D. A. and Frith, J. (1986) The case of the anxious executive: a study from the research clinic, *British Journal of Medicinal Psychology*, 86: 221–33.

This study explored the process of change in a man who was experiencing high levels of anxiety in his work. Mr Trevor was a 42-year-old senior manager who was referred by his GP with depression and anxiety. He was experiencing great stress at work, was unable to concentrate, was very irritable and felt his life was a complete failure. He had become extremely sexually jealous of his wife to such a point that his constant accusations, despite her denials, led to a divorce, although they continued to see each other and could not separate. The work summarized below describes the impact of eight sessions of 'focused psychodynamic therapy' with a female clinical psychologist. Following discussion, ten items capturing his main concerns were jointly derived (see Table 7.2 opposite).

---

It is possible to see from Table 7.2 which sessions appeared to be more helpful than others, what aspects of the problems were particularly helped in each of the sessions and which areas were perceived to change most and least overall. The therapist's views can also be added into such a matrix, which can help to highlight what clients found helpful in comparison to the activities that the therapist had thought were being helpful or otherwise. Importantly, in the first session the client perceived the session as helpful because it gave him hope, whereas the therapist saw the session much more in terms of the content: accounts of the divorce, remorse and loss. This is consistent with much of the psychotherapy research literature which suggests that the non-technical and relational aspects of therapy are paramount in the early stages.

Such an analysis also helps to chart progress for clients and may reveal how some sessions which are experienced as difficult – for example session 2, where there was a discussion of his difficult relations with his mother –

**Table 7.2** Client's perceptions

| Sessions | Possessiveness | Lack of confidence | Depression | Lack of interest | Worry | Tension | Problem delegating | Inability to concentrate | Irritability | Mother problem | Total impact | Helpful events (client's view) | Helpful events (therapist's view) |
|---|---|---|---|---|---|---|---|---|---|---|---|---|---|
| 1 | 0 | +1 | +1 | 0 | 0 | +2 | 0 | 0 | +5 | −1 | +8 | Gave hope that my problems can be helped | Account of events leading to divorce, remorse and loss |
| 2 | 0 | −1 | −1 | 0 | 0 | −1 | 0 | 0 | −6 | +1 | −8 | Realized relationships with others was slightly wrong | History; relations with mother; first link to early life |
| 3 | 0 | 0 | 0 | 0 | 0 | +6 | 0 | +1 | +11 | 0 | +18 | Links made between my attitude to wife and possessiveness of mother to me | Anxiety in the transference; link to parents; death of brother |
| 4 | 0 | 0 | 0 | 0 | 0 | −1 | 0 | −1 | −4 | 0 | −6 | Realized anxiety I feel has always been there | Links between marriage dynamics and early life |
| 5 | 0 | 0 | +1 | 0 | 0 | +4 | +5 | 0 | +3 | −1 | +12 | Realized I must face up to my situation and that I am afraid | Angry part of self; loneliness of the true self |
| 6 | +3 | +2 | +4 | +2 | +2 | +4 | −1 | 0 | +1 | +4 | +21 | Realized I have to make a conscious decision to change | Dilemma of love = needy insecurity, vs. hate = being independent; rage |
| 7 | +3 | +2 | +3 | +3 | +3 | +5 | +2 | +3 | +5 | +2 | +31 | Jigsaw puzzle has clicked into place; somehow links with past events help | Separation issues; creative self blocked by fear of destroying mother |
| 8 | −1 | +3 | 0 | +2 | +2 | +1 | 0 | +4 | +3 | +2 | +16 | Realized extent the past has played in my attitudes to everything | Final session: review of work; D. spontaneously continued links |
| Total | +5 | +7 | +8 | +7 | +7 | 20 | +6 | +7 | +18 | +7 | | | |

may represent important turning points. Consequently, in the third session he made important links between his relationship with his wife and mother, and this was then a very useful session. The chart can reveal which aspects of his problems he experiences as making initial improvements on, such as irritability, and which become amenable to change later in therapy. Such a chart can be employed as a research tool and also as part of an 'ongoing evaluation' of the therapy. This can be completed in a collaborative way with the client and can lead to revisions and changes in emphasis in the formulation and treatment plan. It can also be employed to reveal and

## Research Example 7.9

Bennun, I., Chalkley, A. J. and Donnelly, M. (1987) Research applications of Shapiro's personal questionnaire in marital therapy, *Journal of Family Therapy*, 9: 131–44.

Bennun *et al.* describe examples of employing Shapiro's approach in a piece of research to explore changes in therapy with couples. In one example, Mr and Mrs D were referred for marital therapy following Mrs D's discharge from hospital where she had been treated for symptoms of paranoia and agoraphobia. She had described her marriage as poor and held a belief that her husband had been having an affair. In devising the personal questionnaire the couple identified their main areas of distress as:

1  Mrs D's morbidly jealous thoughts
2  Her fear of leaving the house
3  Their inability to talk about their difficulties
4  Their poor sexual relationship.

In order to develop a system for rating improvements on these areas, they worked with the researcher/therapist to operationalize the problems. For example, it transpired that Mr D was unable, due to his embarrassment, to show his wife any affection in public which she interpreted as lack of interest in her and which was then seen to be expressed as an extreme need for care and attention. This was the problem at its worst (a rating of 3). An improvement was defined when Mrs D sometimes needed a show of care and affection and when Mr D could occasionally demonstrate this in public (rating of 2). A recovery statement was that whenever Mrs D needed such reassurance Mr D could respond whether they were in public or private. Similar clear definitions were derived for the other three areas of difficulty. Using these definitions of the ratings, the couple were able to show how their experience of the intensity of the problems altered as therapy progressed (see Table 7.3).

## Table 7.3

| PQ items (summary) Couple's shared score | Session | | | | | | | | | |
|---|---|---|---|---|---|---|---|---|---|---|
| | 1 | 2 | 3 | 4 | 5 | 6 | 7 | 8 | 9 | 10 |
| Jealousy | 4 | 4 | 3 | 3 | 2 | 1 | 1 | 1 | 2 | 1 |
| Agoraphobia | 4 | 2 | 1 | 1 | 2 | 3 | 3 | 3 | 2 | 2 |
| Communication | 4 | 3 | 3 | 2 | 2 | 1 | 1 | 1 | 1 | 1 |
| Sex | 4 | 4 | 3 | 3 | 2 | 1 | 2 | 1 | 2 | 2 |

*Note:* The scores are summed for each partner so the maximum is $3 \times 2 = 6$ when the problem is worst.

In some cases the couple had difficulty agreeing on their scores and this was employed as a basis for discussion in the sessions. Table 1 suggests that there was some improvement on all four areas fairly rapidly in the sessions though the agoraphobia appears to have taken the longest to ameliorate.

allow a discussion of differences between the client's and therapist's understandings of what is happening. As Rennie's work, discussed earlier in this chapter, suggested, there may be substantial differences between their perceptions.

The construction of the items for a personal questionnaire needs to involve a detailed elaboration of the meanings of the rating employed (see Research Example 7.9). In this case the study examines the experience of couple engaged in therapy. They together agree and draw up relevant items and jointly rate these as the therapy progresses.

This study, as the earlier one, indicates how the process of research and therapy overlap. The process at negotiating the items and agreeing the ratings helps reveal misunderstandings as well as encourages negotiation and clarify which is therapeutically helpful.

## CHAPTER SUMMARY

Case study research offers a comprehensive and detailed analysis of single or multiple therapeutic cases. It can involve both qualitative and quantitative data, which can be employed to *describe* the therapeutic approach, details of procedures and techniques employed and experiences of the therapy. In addition, case studies offer the potential for historical or longitudinal analysis, which together with details of the setting allow causal explanations to be examined and elaborated. They can also serve to indicate what other possible factors need to be considered when scrutiny of the case study reveals that some potentially relevant features of the therapy, such as cultural factors, may have been ignored and could equally, or better, explain the therapy. Psychotherapy case study research has been considered within a broad definition to include what may otherwise be termed case reports, and it has been argued that the distinction between psychotherapy case study research and good case reports may be minimal. This supports the notion of practice based evidence and the reflective scientist–practitioner model of therapy. It has also been suggested that case studies should include the perspectives of clients and, furthermore, needs to be collaborative to constitute 'reflective evidence based practice' and the 'reflective scientist–practitioner' model.

## KEY REFERENCES

Barker, C., Pistrang, N. and Elliott, R. (2002) *Research Methods in Clinical Psychology*, 2nd edn. Chichester: Wiley.

Barlow, D. H. and Hersen, M. (1984) *Single Case Experimental Designs: Strategies for Studying Behaviour Change*. Oxford: Pergamon.

Bem, D. (1994) Evaluating narrative family therapy: using single-system research designs, *Research on Social Work Practice*, 4(3) : 309–25.

Bolger, N., Davis, A. and Rafaeli, E. (2003) Diary methods: capturing life as it is lived, *Annual Review of Psychology*, 54: 579–616.

Morley, S. and Adams, M. (1989) Some simple statistical tests for exploring single-case time-series data, *British Journal of Clinical Psychology*, 28: 1–18.

Sluzki, C. E. and Ransom, D. C. (eds) (1976) *Double Bind: The Foundation of the Communicational Approach to the Family*. New York: Grune and Stratton.

# 8 ■ OBSERVING AND PARTICIPATING

## CHAPTER OVERVIEW

In this chapter we make a case for the importance of observational research in psychotherapy practice and recognize the centrality of observation as a clinical skill. Observational research can play a key role in pilot investigations, in mixed methods studies, in case studies, as part of a triangulation strategy and as the main study. This chapter introduces our model of interpretative observational analysis (IOA) and examines its theoretical roots in the traditions of unstructured observation. IOA relies on participant observation for the collection of data. We describe the four research roles of the participant observer on a continuum of relative involvement and participation. The advantages and disadvantages of each of the research roles are explored. We also pay special attention to the ethical, theoretical and methodological issues of reciprocity in observational research, negotiating access to research participants, consent procedures, reactivity and the impact on the observer, bias, validity and researching within our own organizations. Later, in Chapter 9, we will outline the methodological issues for depth interviewing in research studies and will consider the relationship between interview and observational studies, and how to choose between the methodologies.

## THE CENTRALITY OF OBSERVATION AS A CLINICAL RESEARCH SKILL

Human activity is often characterized as observation, with actions and thoughts grounded in observation of behaviour and consequences in an evolving iterative process. The popularity of Desmond Morris's approach to *People Watching* in the late 1970s and recent 'reality' television like *Big Brother* attests to continuing interest in watching what goes on around us. Attempts at generating lexicons of non-verbal behaviour further testifies to a determined search for an understanding of what it all might mean. For us, this is the stuff of our clinical practice, understanding the reciprocal relationships between talk and action, how they are situated, culturally speaking, and how those reciprocal relationships shift according to the different contexts in which they are played out. Perhaps this curiosity is at the heart of why we chose to enter the field of psychology, and what keeps us motivated.

In our day-to-day clinical work, observation is central, both as a formal and informal process in seeking and gaining feedback. We find ourselves constantly moving between talking and watching, what we do, what our clients do, and what we do together. When thinking about clinical research, we may want to use observational methods, perhaps to further ground an interesting clinical observation, before embarking on a larger study, or because asking directly about our observation might be initially difficult, for example, when observing the play of very young children or fighting amongst young siblings.

In the process of therapy we have to engage in a very complex process wherein we observe our clients – how they look, their posture, facial expressions, tone of voice, movement and so on – and ourselves, as much as we can, and our clients' impact on us, and our impact on them. We use this information to give us ideas about how they are feeling and to make micro clinical decisions about whether to pursue a particular line of questioning, change tack, slow down and so on. We need to observe ourselves – self-observation – both to monitor the process of therapy and our contribution to it. For example, we might ask ourselves: what feelings am I having? How am I talking to this person I am with? What might I look like to them? Not infrequently, for example, we realize that we are mirroring a client by sitting in an identical way or holding a hand to our face just as they are. What does this mean? This is related to the further complex observational task of monitoring our interaction. How are we responding to each other? In working with families we also look for how our response can become part of an interactional pattern. We note with interest here that systemic family therapy training in particular used to emphasize such observational skills, although this has become somewhat marginalized in the face of emphasizing the analysis of talk and narratives. Psychoanalytic training is still one of the areas where observational skills, for example, observing mother–infant interactions, are taught.

In this chapter we want to offer a case for a re-emergence of observational research and recognition of its centrality as a clinical skill. Further, we want to offer a model of interpretative observation as potentially extremely useful in clinical research. In effect, we are suggesting that the kinds of observational activity mentioned above is something that we all do – including clients. Without these skills we could not manage our social interactions. In our view, observation has been neglected in psychotherapy practice and research with the recent 'turn to narrative'. We sometimes wonder if observation challenges some psychotherapy practices because they are exposed to scrutiny. We are systemic psychotherapists, and our training and practice is rooted in live observation, encouraged as part of the process of therapy. Our wish here is to explore the value of psychotherapy observational research, with an emphasis on the use of self through participative methods.

Observation is often used when we have fewer a priori notions, or clear theoretical constructs, to guide us in our enquiry. When choosing observational methods, we may wish to participate in the setting both to collect and generate data for our research questions. At this early stage, we need to make a number of choices, including:

- Decisions about the kinds of observational data we can generate
- What we will look at
- How we will look at it (in terms of using a predetermined coding scheme or not) and even whether we know what we are looking for
- What settings to choose
- How our immersion in the setting might shape what we see and do not see
- How we act and respond
- How we set about making relationships in the setting
- How we record our observations
- How we negotiate our departure

## INTERPRETATIVE OBSERVATIONAL ANALYSIS

### The analysis of observational data

Typically, observational research methods have come to focus on tightly structured forms of observation. This can involve the use of observational systems which involve training of observers to generate good levels of inter-rater reliability in the use of the system. Perhaps one of the best known systems has been Bales' (1950) analysis of group dynamics. In the field of attachment theory, there is the systematic observation of separation and of reunion behaviour in the Strange Situation paradigm. At the other end of the spectrum, there are the participative methods of ethnography which do not require the use of such systematic observational systems but do involve detailed reflections and interpretations based on an immersion in the area of interest. (See Fig. 8.1.)

We want to suggest that there is an intermediate form of observation that can utilize structure and also interpretation. In fact this 'interpretative observation' is typically what people do in their daily lives: we employ our natural abilities to integrate a wide range of observational information to give meaning to what the participants are doing, what their intentions are and where the interpersonal process between them may be heading and what it means. Frequently, we do this by assigning behaviour to interpersonal episodes, for example, an argument, teasing, apology, justification and so on. This idea is supported further by Heider's (1958) experiments which revealed that even when people are asked to watch a film consisting of the random movement of inanimate shapes they invariably assigned meanings in episodes and intentions to these shapes: they turned the random movements into a story with a plot and drama. So we want to suggest that a reflexive use of this natural ability to integrate our observations into a meaningful analysis could help to revitalize the use of observation in psychotherapy settings. In effect, it is giving permission for clinicians to do what they already do quite well, namely observe the behaviour of our clients and ourselves.

## The theoretical roots of interpretative observational analysis

However we may collect our observational data, we shall need to analyse and make sense of it, in pursuit of either problem setting and/or problem solving (Wolcott, 1990). Data can be collected and analysed concurrently, or analysis can be withheld for later consideration, as far as that is possible. For example, we can record sequential behavioural descriptions in narrative

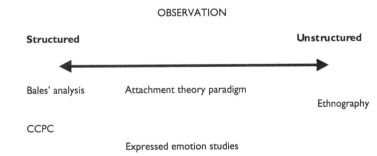

**Figure 8.1**   The dimensional nature of observation

form, where we interpret motivations and intent, as an attempt to explore the relationship between latent and manifest activity, or we may try to withhold such interpretations, when observing within an undertheorized area of activity. The value for us in conducting observational psychotherapy research is that we can utilize our clinical experiences and understandings in the analytic activity. As systemic practitioners ourselves, we would use concepts derived from systemic theory, ethnography and social constructionism.

It is of interest to note that the family systemic therapies grew out of the research interests of the grandparents of family therapy. For example, Bateson and the MRI project produced some rich research on communication (Watzlawick *et al.*, 1967); Minuchin produced research evidence to support his model of the dynamics of families linked to psychosomatic processes (Minuchin *et al.*, 1978); and the Milan team attempted to explore systematically therapeutic strategies for the treatment of family members with a diagnosis of anorexia nervosa and schizophrenia (Palazzoli, 1974). The aims of this early clinical oriented observational research in the family therapy field were to:

- develop causal explanations, such as how patterns of actions over time can give rise to other problems
- develop typologies, such as what family interaction patterns were associated with different types of problems
- develop appropriate therapeutic interventions, such as models of clinical practice that indicate where and how to intervene in sequences of behaviour to disrupt problem-maintaining sequences of action.

The theoretical assumptions that influenced some of these early observations included a mix of behaviourism, psychodynamic theories and systemic theories. Theories and philosophies move on and, admittedly, some of the early research could be seen as 'expert' and perhaps not always aware of the need for a political/historical analysis of the interests of family therapy. However, there may be a danger of 'throwing the baby out with the bath water', for example, when we ignore the brilliant observations of the multi-faceted nature of communication to concentrate our interests solely on language and narrative. The emphasis in early systemic research and practice on observation and the analysis of non-verbal behaviour, patterning and actions, is arguably, still central to the contribution of systemic therapy. Interestingly, such observations are a cornerstone of developmental psychology.

The legacy of this early work is contained in a set of concepts about communication, context and internal states that guide our interpretative observational activity. These concepts are worth revisiting here:

- Meanings are co-constructed through communication.
- All actions are potential communications.
- Communication is multifaceted.
- Communication is both verbal and non-verbal, and may be consistent or contradictory.

- Communication is multilevelled, with layers of meanings contextually embedded within relationships, scripts and cultural discourses.
- Language is one form of communication and is not totally privileged.
- Communications/actions are given meaning by the context.
- Context and actions are reciprocally related.
- Participants and observers have reciprocal roles in interactions.
- To engage in interaction and/or to observe it involves making inferences about internal states. For example, 'why' is X acting, speaking, feeling in a particular way?

### Interpretative observational analysis

IOA (interpretative observational analysis) is interpretative because as psychotherapy researchers we are making interpretations about the meanings of people's behaviours, actions and sequences of actions. Central to this is that we are making inferences about the possible intentions and choices that people are making. The choices may be more or less conscious. The interpretations are based in our own belief systems and theoretical frameworks of understandings. These are, in turn, shaped by dominant social discourses and the use of language. It is interesting to note that our experience of ourselves and of others and our relationships can be profoundly shaped by the language system we use to express ourselves (Burck, 2005). However, in our work we are trying to get as close as we can to the possible understandings that participants hold about their own and each other's actions and choices and their awareness of the patterns of interaction in which they are involved.

IOA is observational because we are interested in both verbal and non-verbal actions. These can be observed as individual actions and patterns of actions. A core interest for us is in mutually constructed patterns of actions. Underpinning this is our understanding that actions are seen as constructing patterns and also that patterns construct individual actions. Observational activity within an IOA framework focuses on actions, feelings and thoughts as the basic units of analysis, both of the participants and also of the observer. The observation can involve taking observational notes, the analysis of video-tape, retrospective note-taking, the use of a reflective diary, and collaborative analysis, such as, comprehensive process analysis and interpersonal process recall (Elliott, 1986). (For a description of video-tape or audio-tape sequences of therapy interactions, see Chapter 9.) The observation can be primarily of individuals, couples, families, groups, teams and of the observer.

Analytic activity within IOA involves analysis, synthesis and reflexivity. A variety of possible systems of analysis can be used, such as expressed emotion coding, structural theory analysis, Bales' small group observational categories and levels of engagement. Synthesis focuses our activity on making sense of the observations by weaving together the different levels of analysis utilizing the observer's explicit and implicit frameworks. A reflexive stance promotes the use of self in making sense of our observations: we actively refer to our own frameworks and beliefs, both experiential and theoretical. Reflexivity in our work requires us to actively reflect on the assumptions, beliefs and explanatory frameworks that shape our analysis and synthesis, and which crucially filter our idiosyncratic interpretation of theory. We make use of research supervision and consultation and keep a reflective diary or research journal to aid the processes of analysis and synthesis.

## THE SOCIAL ROLES OF THE PARTICIPANT OBSERVER

In this section we outline the participative roles of the participant observer, the method of choice when our observations are likely to be less structured and we are more interested in exploring a phenomenon. We shall discuss some of the dilemmas and solutions that can be experienced within each of the participative roles.

Participant observation as a research method can be characterized along a number of dimensions:

- The relative involvement and participation of the observer in the activity under scrutiny.
- The degree of inference and interpretation used by the observer, both in making sense of others' responses and their own responses, and their interaction over time.
- The confidentiality of the observation process.
- Concealment of the observational activity.

Junker (1972) described the social roles of the participant observer along a continuum, ranging from the complete participant, to participant as observer, observer as participant, and complete observer (see Fig. 8.2). Junker anticipated that any participant observer working in naturalistic settings would find themselves moving in and out of these roles, along the continuum of relative involvement, even though they might try to adopt as primary, one of these social roles. These roles are described in greater detail

| The complete participant | The participant as observer |
|---|---|
| Rosenhan 'On being sane in insane places' | Goffman's work |
| Festinger 'When prophecy fails' | Jane Gilgun |
| The observer as participant | The complete observer |
| Vetere and Gale | Jane Gilgun |
| Early MRI studies | Michael Argyle's work |

**Figure 8.2**  Junker's categories of observational rule

in Vetere and Gale (1987). Thus the interpretative activity, possible within each role, varies along the following dimension:

complete   participant   observer as   complete
participant   →   as observer   →   participant   →   observer

High level of                              Structured reflection, i.e.
interpretation. Personal          interpretation structured by
and socio-political                   'objective' epistemology
reflectivity need:
'subjective' epistemology

Our choice of method of recording will reflect our interpretative activity. So, for example, we may wish to keep interpretation to a minimum during the observation process, by recording behavioural, sequential narrative descriptions, which we subject to later analysis, such as coding, theme analysis, or theoretical analysis, which includes more or less inferential activity. Alternatively, we may record our observations using interpretations at the time, so that analysis has already begun, overtly, while the observer is still in the field. In addition, we have the choice of using more structured observational tools, such as pre-determined coding schemes, with the participant as observer, the observer as participant and the complete observer roles. An example can be found in the 'levels of engagement' research, conducted some years ago, in residential homes for older frail people, or for people with profound learning difficulties. Observers would record every instance of engagement between a resident and a member of staff, how long it lasted and who initiated it. Such observations can be subject to reliability studies. Although engagement is an apparently simple notion, it can be quite powerful in helping service providers to critique their own practice and to think about how and where to improve levels of engagement.

## The complete participant

The complete participant is totally involved with the group of persons under study, and conceals their observational activity from the group. This allows the observer to act as a member of an 'in-group', perhaps sharing private information that would not have been disclosed to an identifiable observer. The advantage is that the observer develops an intimate acquaintance with a particular social role and has access to private worlds, which potentially provide rich data. However, the disadvantages are great. Ethically, our codes of conduct disallow observation without the consent of the participants, and we would be open to accusations of spying. Alongside this, there is the problem for the observer of subsuming their own identity in order to join the group and, subsequently, of how they manage alliance formations within the group. Opportunities for observation outside the 'in-group' may be limited. An example can be found in the Festinger *et al.* study, *When Prophecy Fails* (1956). Two researchers joined a small group of people who predicted the end of the world as 'believers'.

They wished to observe what would happen within the group when the world did not end! This extended study spawned the theory of cognitive dissonance.

## The participant as observer

The participant as observer already has or takes on a meaningful social role within the group under study. The role is characterized by relative involvement with the group. For example, Jane Gilgun (1994) observed her clinical multidisciplinary team colleagues' decision-making processes, whilst acting as a member of the team herself. Observational activity is not wholly concealed, but observers often find the group members evaluate them on the basis of their group participation rather than on their status as an observer.

The advantages include familiarity with a particular role within the group, with increased understanding of group processes from this more subjective and sympathetic position. There is relative freedom to observe within the group, although observational activity may be constrained by the demands of the particular role adopted within the group. Disadvantages include limited access to some private information, with more time and energy spent participating than observing! Other examples can be found in William Whyte's work, *Street Corner Society: The Social Structure of an Italian Slum* (1955).

## The observer as participant

The observer as participant joins the group with the expressed intention to observe. Their role as observer is characterized by relative detachment from the group under study, with their objective and empathic positioning emphasized. Advantages include access to a wide range of material, even private information if it becomes known that the observer can maintain anonymity for the group members. The observer is in many ways freer to ask questions in this role, unrestrained by the role demands of participation. The observer as participant is less active than the participant as observer. The latter carries responsibility to participate within the group and initiates activity, whereas the former tends to be more reactive to the initiatives of the group members. Disadvantages of this role can include constraints on confidentiality when reporting and a sense of marginality – the observer is *in* the world of the group members, but not *of* their world. The observer has to be mindful of the need to maintain a degree of even-handedness or neutrality relative to internal alliances and factions within the group. This can be an emotionally demanding task, particularly if the observational study separates the observer from their own social group and sources of social support and affirmation of personal identity. An example of this role can be found in the work of Arlene Vetere, in her ecological studies of family life (Vetere and Gale, 1987).

### The complete observer

The role of the complete observer is characterized by detachment from the group under study, with no direct contact with group members during the observational work. This is approximated in some clinical work, when activity is viewed from behind a one-way screen, or in a field setting, with non-declared observation, such as observing rituals of greeting and farewell at major international airports. It is possible to use pre-prepared coding schemes, and to subject them to intra-coder and inter-coder reliability studies. Another example can be found in viewing video-tapes of clinical work. There are no risks of observational reactivity, but the observer is never *in* the situation, with no opportunity to share in the experiential world of the participants.

## GAINING ACCESS TO RESEARCH PARTICIPANTS

All field researchers need to negotiate access to research participants with individuals, within organizational structures, with different levels of seniority and influence. The notional 'gatekeepers' of our research activity have more or less power to facilitate access. In our experience it is helpful to have done your homework first, researching and understanding the roles and responsibilities of those who can facilitate your entry to your chosen research site. It might be the case that a senior manager, for example, might give permission for you to interview employees, but less senior staff might actually have the responsibility for setting up meetings between you and your potential research participants. Understanding both the formal and informal networks of communication within the organization in which you want to carry out your research is essential. It is often a matter of knowing who to talk to, and who has influence, alongside the more formal procedures of obtaining permission. It is helpful to know beforehand whether cooperation might be likely, before embarking on a process of negotiating access, which can often be very time consuming and lengthy.

Reciprocity is a key issue. What is in it for the research participant? Why should they cooperate with your research endeavour? Not all researchers are in a position to remunerate their research participants. It may be possible to organize a small token of appreciation but more usually, a field researcher will offer to give of their time to the organization. Presentation of research findings in the form of a booklet, or a talk, will go a long way to acknowledging the debt to the group. Research ethics committees will often require researchers to present their findings to the group studied. The question of reciprocity raises other questions of motivations to participate in field research and to open oneself to outside scrutiny. This will be addressed in more detail below.

In conducting observational research we gain access to private worlds and private information. We can develop quite intense relationships within our research roles that may not continue beyond the observational study. We may find ourselves in conflict with the wish to retain a relative degree of involvement and a pull to get involved with the group under study, where we are asked to give our opinions or even take action around potentially sensitive and conflictual areas. We may be exposed directly to group conflict and asked to take sides. We may hear views and opinions expressed which we personally find distasteful. Clearly, as observers we carry a duty of care and we are bound by our code of conduct, such that we could not ignore direct harm or risk of harm. (See Bussell, 1994, and Bussell *et al.*, 1995, for a detailed discussion of these issues.) However, much of the data we hear and see do not fall into this category but do require us to make decisions quickly about how we respond without alienating group members whilst trying to maintain our relative status as an observer within the group. Such a task is not suited to us all. It is important to find out how you might react to these role demands when under pressure. For example:

- How has your resilience and sense of humour been tested in the past?
- Are you comfortable with not having answers and remaining open to possibilities?
- Are you in the habit of reflecting on yourself and the situation you are in?
- Do you keep in mind the distinction between your own assumptions and those of others?
- How do you manage closeness and distance in relationships while remaining interpersonally sensitive?

Thus it is helpful when considering an intense observational study to first pilot the method with a willing group of volunteers, such as a group of colleagues, who will give you straightforward feedback and help with the debriefing and reflecting process afterwards.

Ethically speaking, we try to negotiate consent to participate in an observational study as best we can. We keep the following issues in mind at all times, and regularly discuss them in research supervision:

- What will happen to the observational data subsequently?
- Who will get to see it?
- How will anonymity be managed?
- How can confidentiality be managed with publication and wider presentation of the findings in mind?

Consent is predicated on anonymity, in our experience. Although we try to ensure informed consent, we could argue that living under the constant scrutiny of an observer is hard to imagine until it has actually been experienced. Research ethics committees' consent procedures require participants to sign a consent form, which guarantees the possibility for withdrawal at any stage of the study. It is perhaps harder for a participant to withdraw from a longer observational study, where relationships are developed and fears of letting people down may predominate, as compared to withdrawal from an interview, say, or a brief experimental study. As discussed above, the different social roles of the participative observer can vary in terms of the relative activity of the observer within the group under study. Whether the observer takes on a more active role, initiating activity, or a more passive, reactive role, the observer can be an instigator of change. It is of moral interest to consider what might have happened within the group had the observer not been present. Clearly, we can never know this, but if research is intervention into people's lives, the presence of a reacting observer will have an effect within the group.

The observer needs to invest energy into maintaining the observational roles, possibly at some personal cost, and to negotiate a planned withdrawal from the group under study. In many ways this has parallels with our clinical roles, where we keep in mind the termination of clinical work during the processes of engagement and middle therapy. If the observer has spent significant time with the group under observation, they may have developed a sense of commitment to the group and may wish to keep in touch subsequently. Research supervision is helpful in identifying responsibilities to the group under study and the less helpful breaches of roles and overstepping of responsibilities within the group.

# SPECIAL PROBLEMS OF PARTICIPANT OBSERVATION

Participant observation raises some special problems, such as reactivity, the bias of the observer, the validity of the findings and researching within our own organizations.

## Reactivity

The problem for observational research is that the activity under observation is changed by the act of observation, or as Stapp, a quantum physicist, put it: 'The observed system is required to be isolated in order to be defined, yet interacting in order to be observed' (1971). Thus observers are not thought to be separate from what they study, and their ordinary knowledge about people and relationships and their personal values are understood to affect their research activity. As an interactive process, observation and thus observational data can be thought of as an emergent property of the process. There is much debate in the observational literature about the nature and magnitude of reactivity. For us, reactivity depends upon the context of the observation and who is present. Reactivity effects are an important source of working hypotheses. For example, we need to ask why some forms of reactivity effects occur, such as strong attention seeking behaviour from some people towards the observer compared with others, or whether reactivity effects indicate we might be paying attention to less relevant factors (London and Thorngate, 1981).

Observational data are rich in quality and may be gathered under three conditions: explicit observation, as agreed with the participants; inadvertent display; and that offered in intimate moments, usually within dyadic interaction.

Observation is both an intervention into the lives of the observed and an intervention into the life of the observer, in a mutual process of influence and change. A participant observer living or working with a social group is often obliged to self-disclose personal information. The observational work may last for days. The observer cannot 'hide' behind the administration of a questionnaire, or within a semi-structured interview, which may only last one hour. The observer may become a confidant(e), or may be seen as a guest and friend as well as a watcher. The various roles might merge, both conferring power and stripping power.

## Bias

Bias is assumed here to be part of all research activity regardless of the methods used or their philosophical underpinnings. Perception can be considered an active and interpretative process, so that observers will be responding on the basis of their own preconceptions and experiences. At the worst, we could say that observers will only see what they expect to see! We are always researching within and across subcultural groupings, and sometimes across wider cultures. Celia Falicov's (1998) idea of cultural borderlands is helpful when thinking about predisposition to bias and motivated perception. She argues that each of us is raised in, and living in, a plurality of cultural subgroups that have a multiplicity of influences. As we move within and between these subgroups, she would say that the degree of cultural influence varies with the degree of contact with each grouping. So, as observers and researchers, the way we think, feel and behave is shaped by cultural themes and, similarly, we reinterpret, reproduce and constitute those themes in our day-to-day living (Krause, 1995).

Observers have a responsibility to describe behaviour and use of language and to use language to interpret behaviour. The observer's language may be inadequate to the task of describing complex human interaction and different observers may well differ in the language they use. However, as clinicians we have been trained to try to identify and appreciate our own values and preconceptions. Continuing supervision and consultation helps attune us to our own perceptual biases and how our responses to roles and role structures may not always be consciously determined. The use of more than one observer, and asking observers to keep a personal journal to record their reflections and responses when observing, can aid in the early identification of preconceived assumptions about what 'is' or 'should be' in the context of human activity.

## Validity

Validity is discussed at length in Chapter 10. We wish to comment here on the problems for naturalistic data. Naturalistic data are not replicable in the quantitative sense, and some commentators might wish to dismiss such data as anecdotal. However, we would argue that although replicability may not be feasible, single observations, supported with strategies of corroboration, can be acceptable. Similarly, some behaviours may be more readily observed than others and some observational coding schemes may be reliable. But if we argue that to some extent each individual's view of the world is unique and in some respects inconsistent with that of others, the problem for us is to establish to what extent there is a shared social reality, or whose reality it is (Laing and Esterson, 1964). When considering several different points of view simultaneously, we may not be able to capture a communal view without damaging the integrity of individual views. We offer a range of validity strategies in Chapter 10 that seek to sample a number of views and offer a grounding for naturalistic data studies.

## Researching within our own organizations

When clinicians choose to conduct research with their own clients, or within their own organization, they may face more externally expressed doubts about the validity of their research or their credibility as researchers. The participant observer who chooses to research their own organization needs to find a position, akin to 'being a stranger in one's own land'. On the one hand, they are in a very privileged position, because they have personal and shared experience of the organization, its members, its codes of conduct and ways of working. On the other hand, they risk taking much for granted, operating from within their own biases, and they risk alienating colleagues when making overt what might have been taken for granted if it cuts across perceived vested interests. And, of course, they have to continue working in their organization with their colleagues once their research is complete. Many of the projects we supervise fall into this category – for example, small-scale psychotherapy process studies with one or two clients, case studies with one or two clients, small-scale service evaluations and user surveys – and all involve either direct observation or an interpretative observation component. The task is to produce research that capitalizes on the researcher's special knowledge and understanding of the organization or therapy process, whilst at the same time not losing sight of these external credibility issues when planning the research.

Thus researching from the 'insider' perspective raises some interesting ethical and methodological issues. Anonymity in reporting the study findings needs special attention, particularly when reporting internally, publishing the findings or lodging the research report in the library as part of a professional qualification process. Obviously small samples can be collated and analysed collectively as a way of protecting anonymity. When researching the single case, so to speak, a different strategy needs to be considered. The research participant(s) can give consent to dissemination again, in a two-part manner: once the findings have been produced, or as part of the validation strategy, they can be asked to produce their own analysis of the data or to comment on the researcher's analysis.

Informed consent to participation in research is always fraught, in that we could say we do not know what we are consenting to until we have experienced it. All ethical committees require researchers to make it very clear that research participants can withdraw from the study at any time, without giving a reason and without it affecting their treatment if they are clinical participants. However, when researching with our own clients, or within our own teams, it may be harder to withdraw, for reasons of loyalty and not wanting to let our colleagues down. Where this happens, such processes can sit uncomfortably between coercion and consent.

Boundary issues need some careful thought when researching our own organizations. The researcher/clinician carries a dual role, at least. There may be a conflict of interest within the two roles that needs careful discussion with team members, particularly if the clinician's role carries authority and power. An external consultant to the research process can help provide a safety net for concerns about the impact of researching potentially sensitive internal issues. Having said all the above, the benefits of researching our own therapy and in our own organizations can be profound: they contribute to learning, both for ourselves, our practice and our organizations, when we try to understand and confront our own and others' assumptions and lived experiences, grounded in our day-to-day interactions. Thus we can be said to be working in learning organizations.

## APPROACHES TO STRUCTURED OBSERVATION

When describing structured quantitative observation, Elliott (1991) put forward a five-stage process of decision making. We shall draw on his framework in describing the tasks of structured observation.

The first stage is the perspective of the observation study when the point of view of the person doing the observation tasks needs to be made clear. Is the researcher a trained observer, for example, trained in the reliable use of a coding scheme? Or an expert participant, such as a psychotherapist or psychotherapy supervisor? Or an index participant, such as a psychotherapy client, or supervisee?

The second stage is the focus of the observation, such as: which element of the behavioural process is studied? Is it the client or client system (index participant), the psychotherapist or their agency (expert participant), or the rated quality of their relationship (interaction of index and expert participants)?

The third stage involves the decision around what kind of behaviour or process variable(s) are to be studied – the aspect of behaviour.

- Content, or what is said, meant or expressed (as ideas or themes).
- Action/intention, or what is done by what is said, such as, actions or behaviours carried out by participants, including intentions, tasks and response modes.
- Style, or how it is done, said or expressed, such as duration, frequency or intensity, mood, interpersonal manner, paralinguistic and non-verbal behaviour, and vocal quality.
- Quality, or how well is it said, done or expressed, such as accuracy, skilfulness, and appropriateness.

Stage four is unit level or selected useful units of study. This involves the decision around what level or resolution the process is studied. According to Elliott (1991), there are seven aspects to this:

1 Idea unit, such as a sentence, or single expressed idea
2 Interaction unit, such as a speaking turn, an action by one participant in response to the action of another participant

3  Topic or task unit, such as an episode, a series of actions or speaking turns organized by participation in one task within an occasion
4  Scene unit, or occasion, a time-limited interaction between two people
5  Interpersonal unit, such as the relationship between two people
6  Institution unit, or organization, such as a system of relationships organized towards specific goals located in setting, such as a clinic
7  Self unit or person, which includes a person's relatively stable set of beliefs, characteristics and history of self, other and organizational involvement.

The final stage is the sequential phase, or decisions about what happened before, during or after the unit of process. This is made up of:

■ Context, or antecedents, such as what led up to a process, like previous speaking turns, behaviours
■ Process or behaviours, such as the particular process that is observed at a given level or unit
■ Effects, or consequences, such as the sequelae of a unit of process, like psychotherapy outcomes.

Once the level of observation has been decided, a decision on the use of a coding scheme versus developing a coding scheme needs to be made. This is determined by whether the study intends to explore or generate hypotheses. Coding schemes have been developed for micro coding, such as the occurrence of smiling during an activity, or for macro coding, such as rated expressed emotion during an interview, where categories are pre-determined. Automatic devices permit time sampling and event sampling. Observers/raters need to be trained to achieve reassuring levels of reliability; usually correlations of 0.8 are acceptable. Such procedures minimize inter-action with research participants and reduce reactivity effects. Reliability studies usually seek both intra-observer reliability and inter-observer reliability, as well as reliability of the coding scheme across time.

## KEY REFERENCES

Goffman, E. (1959) *The Presentation of Self in Everyday Life*. Garden City, NY: Doubleday-Anchor.
Goffman, E. (1961) *Asylums*. Chicago: Aldine.
Vetere, A. and Gale, T. (1987) *Ecological Studies of Family Life*. Chichester: Wiley.

# 9 INTERVIEW METHODOLOGY

## CHAPTER OVERVIEW

This chapter addresses the questions of when, why and how we would choose to interview our research participants. As clinicians we know that interviewing involves a complex set of decisions and skills. We explore the context, content and process of interviewing and pay attention to the practicalities of planning and setting up an interview study.

The chapter addresses the special problems and dilemmas involved in conjoint interviewing, as it tends to receive less attention in the research methods literature than one-to-one interviewing methods. We discuss the collaborative and flexible use of focus groups, the Delphi method and Interpersonal Process Recall as structured forms of conjoint depth interviewing. In addition, we explore questionnaire design as a highly structured method of interviewing. Our discussion of the various approaches to interviewing includes aspects of the analysis of interview data (see Chapter 4) and how our approach to interpretative observational analysis (see Chapter 8) can inform the analysis of the context, content and process of the interview. We close the chapter with a detailed exploration of the relationship between observation and interviewing as psychotherapy research activities and offer help with how to decide when to choose depth interviewing or observation, or when to use them in a complementary manner.

# SETTING UP AN INTERVIEW STUDY

## Why choose to interview?

As psychotherapist researchers, we may wish to explore the meaning of an experience for our clients. Typically then, researchers will decide to *ask* people about their experiences and their understanding of how they attribute meaning to events and relationships, and how such meaning changes over time and in different contexts. In this way, our analysis would attempt to stay close to our participants' meanings as we understand and interpret them. This presumes people can monitor their own behaviour and give an account of it (Harre and Secord, 1972). Similarly, we might be interested in how people explain or justify their actions, or what ideas, held culturally, could be said to influence their accounts. Again we would ask people to talk to us about their understandings, but our analysis would focus more on our 'observations' and interpretation of the interplay of larger ideas in their interview transcripts. Harre and Secord suggest that people's accounts do not have to be accepted at face value – they can be negotiated. Since the perspective of the interviewer is likely to be different from that of the interviewee, this divergence forms the basis on which they negotiate a shared account.

As psychotherapists we are trained in the use of interview methods as one medium of collecting information and ideas, and as part of the vehicle for developing a therapeutic relationship. Transferring our clinical skills to research interviewing is paradoxically both easy and problematic, as we discuss elsewhere. What we wish to highlight here, is our enormous advantage as clinicians in our ability to develop and discard hypotheses, in our reservoir of ordinary knowledge about people and relationships and in our ability to question in a sensitively attuned manner, to match our observations with what we are being told and to know when to stop asking questions. We offer these thoughts in contrast to the findings of some studies, which purport to show a marked reluctance on the part of clinicians either to conduct research or to participate in research (Sandberg *et al.*, 2002). Reasons often cited include lack of time, outside limitations, concerns about clients' well-being, and importantly, from our point of view, a lack of understanding of research methods and research process. It is the last reason we wish to challenge.

## Setting up an interview

Interviewing is a common method of data collection and is used widely to elicit people's views in a range of contexts, including psychotherapy research. In fact, it could be suggested that within psychotherapy research it is fast becoming the most common method of data collection. This could carry risks of what might be called 'the taken for granted', since interviewing is so akin to everyday conversation, even though turn taking might be somewhat more formalized. Just as we write about the need to be a stranger in your own land when doing observational work, so we would suggest that an attitude of curiosity while interviewing is not only important, but needs to be actively encouraged and maintained (Cecchin, 1987). Research diaries, research supervision and consultation, can all be contexts in which we ask ourselves, what is taken for granted in this account? Despite the proliferation of guides to interviewing, there is little psychological theory of direct relevance to the practice and conduct of interviews that integrates the intrapersonal and interpersonal experiences of the interviewee and the interviewer. We would suggest that psychotherapeutic theories of listening, Goffman's (1959) work on the presentation of self in everyday life and systemic approaches to understanding connection, relationships and feedback provide a helpful framework for thinking about the process of research interviewing.

In deciding to conduct an interview study, we need to think about the process of the interview itself and our responsibilities to our research participants. An interview can be described as proceeding through a number of stages: initiation and preparation; conduct; purpose; and consequences of the interview, for both interviewer and the interviewed (Wicks, 1982). A situational analysis helps to identify the important aspects of the interview situation for those involved, and the meaning and effects of those aspects.

### Initiation and preparation

Preparation for the interviews needs time and resources. Our planning is based around our research aims and what we hope to achieve, and as outlined in Chapter 2, seeking and securing permission for participation can be lengthy and needs thought. Clearly, we need to seek ethical permission to proceed with our study from the relevant bodies, for example, the local research ethics committees, when interviewing within a client group. Preliminary visits to potential participants, or 'gatekeepers', may need to be made to explain our work and our intentions and set the scene for the interviews. When working across cultural groups, we need to invest a lot of time meeting with community leaders and key people in the community to introduce ourselves and to explore the vexed question of reciprocity: in what ways will research participation benefit the community and not be exploitative, in that the research will only benefit the researcher? During such preliminary visits, our research aims will often shift to encompass local community interests.

A timetable needs to be planned that allows for this preliminary work, for conducting the interviews, transcribing and editing the interviews, and the analysis of the interviews. A decision needs to be made about how to record the interviews. Usually interviews are audio-taped. If possible, the use of a video suite is preferred because of superior sound recording. We have lost count of the number of student research projects we have supervised where the sound quality of the recorded interview is so poor that it cannot be transcribed. It is so important to test the sound quality before starting the interview and at times during the interview, even though we might fear this interrupts the flow of conversation. In some circumstances our interviewees will not consent to recording, and we need to negotiate whether we can take notes during the interview, or immediately afterwards. Clearly, problems of memory will predominate at this time, and anxiety that we might be so focused on remembering what is said that we do not pay sufficient attention to facilitating the process of the interview. Under such circumstances we advise a style of interviewing that identifies and reviews key themes or interests during the interview, to aid recall, and to ensure we are appropriately representing the issues for our informants, or we have understood their position for a more discursive reading. Transcription is a lengthy business! We estimate that a one-hour interview takes ten hours to transcribe. We always encourage those we supervise to transcribe at least one to three interviews themselves if at all possible, even though someone else might take on the bulk of the task. This facilitates an immersion in the data, so crucial for qualitative methods of analysis, whilst allowing the process of the interview, and thus the observations of the interviewer, to come forth in the text. Editing back into the transcript the non-verbal aspects of the interview, as remembered, provides a richer text for subsequent analysis. This editing can be done by the interviewer subsequently if the interviews have been transcribed by someone else.

## Conduct

The conduct of the interview can be thought of as having two components: the context of the interview and the process of the interview.

We always recommend piloting an interview schedule, and experiencing the process of interviewing, as part of the study itself. Pilot interviewing can be an early stage of the research, as in a grounded theory study, or it can be phase one of a larger study that seeks to ground and validate the research questions before moving on to a larger survey, for example. In our view, pilot data are data, whether they are pooled in the larger set of interview data or treated separately. We say this because we often meet clinician researchers who fear that their pilot data are in some way invalid and should be discarded, particularly when pilot interviewing was conducted to help refine the research questions for subsequent interviews. We see this as part of the natural history of research enquiry. The work done in honing our research question is as interesting as the work done around the research questions.

In terms of the *context* of the interview, we need to decide where it might be held, whether we can protect against interruptions, provide some privacy and attend to our interviewees' comfort. We have supervised interview based research where the interviews have taken place in public places, such as cafes, restaurants and parks, because informants do not want others to know they are participating in a study that is politically and/or personally sensitive, for example in Charity Tawodzera's (personal communication) study on women's narratives about the development of sexual identity and orientation beliefs and practices. Similarly, interviews might take place in people's homes, where rules of social behaviour for guests can predominate and where we might have little control over interruptions. It is harder to be assertive in someone else's home, when you are offered the comfortable chair, but find your knees around your chin, or the family dog takes a constant interest in your groin, and the neighbour's children run in and out. Hence planning can aid in anticipating some of these (humorous with hindsight) dilemmas and how we might agree with participants the conditions for privacy and comfort.

Similarly, when thinking of comfort and privacy for our participants, we need to think of the potential for distress. Small-scale qualitative studies in under-theorized areas of enquiry will often rely on methods of adventitious sampling and snowballing techniques. So we start where we can, with whomever will speak to us who represents some aspects of the issue that is of interest to us. Our ethical committee permission will have involved us in articulating clearly how we will deal with instances of distress during interviews, by assurances that we will stop the interview, and check if the interviewee would like to withdraw; how we will offer support information about appropriate counselling services; and if the interviewee is a client in therapy, how we will liaise, if appropriate, with the clinician. This is fine and proper, but sometimes, the nature and depth of the distress that can be evoked during the interview is a surprise both to the interviewee and to the interviewer. AV supervised a project exploring parents' concerns for their children's well-being and development, where one of the parents had experienced enduring mental health problems and had extensive contact with adult mental health services and their child had been referred to a child and adolescent mental health service. It was hard to secure a research sample in this project for a number of organizational reasons, so the early sampling depended on word-of-mouth recommendation within local services. The first person interviewed had overcome her mental health difficulties many years ago and believed she would be fine when exploring her retrospective concerns for her children. To her surprise, the interview re-evoked grief and regret that she thought she had long since understood and processed. The interviewer was an experienced therapist herself and was able to offer comfort and help process the impact of the research question. The interviewer was reassured that her participant was sufficiently recovered to walk back out on to the street, and she followed her up afterwards, as you might expect. But what the interviewer did not anticipate was the effect of her participant's distress on her. The impact was so strong she nearly abandoned her research aim at that point.

The *process* of the interview reflects the nature and quality of our listening, our ability to be flexible in response to what develops and our clarity around our aims. As described elsewhere in this chapter, the process also strongly reflects how we communicate and integrate verbal with non-verbal information. The demand characteristics within an interview may well be communicated non-verbally, such as attempts by the participant to please the interviewer and search out their 'real' agenda and the management of 'self-presentation' and 'defensive' positioning, for both researcher and researched. The process of the interview interweaves with the content of the interview in a mutually complementary way. We hope we have made it clear that understanding this interplay is as important to the research aims as the analysis of the content of the interview transcripts. Goffman (1959) observed that impressions are 'given off' as well as 'managed'. Clinically trained interviewers are adept at listening to what people choose to say, at helping people say what they otherwise cannot say without help, and in detecting what people may not want to talk about. The tension between what people say and what they might be observed to do can be explored within an interview format, both by asking people to be reflexive about this dilemma and by comparing and contrasting our observational data on the process of the interview with the interview transcript. Our approach to interpretative observational analysis, described in detail in Chapter 8, can form the context for a process analysis of the conduct and consequences of an interview.

## Purpose

The *content* of the interview will in part be determined by the format of the questioning, which is determined by the purpose of the research. Interviews are often described on a continuum from structured, through semi-structured, to unstructured, depending on the degree of standardization required in the questioning. Interview questions will usually be developed on the basis of personal and professional experience and preliminary reading of the literature. The suitability and validity of the questions are often piloted, within pre-pilot consultation with colleagues and clients, and pilot interviews, where explicit feedback may be sought on the intelligibility and relevance of the questions. Questions can be open, closed and scaled. Pitfalls can include asking questions that are overlong, leading and biased in one direction. Probe questions can be asked to explore topics further. In narrative or life history interviewing, the interviewer may open by asking a question of invitation to recount biographical material.

Grounded theorists use a form of interviewing they call 'directed conversations'. They recognize that the conversational aspect of the interview is necessary to build rapport that at the same time encourages disclosure. (As we saw in Chapter 4, a grounded theory study progresses with the aid of theoretical sampling and constant comparison.) Their ethnographic approach to interviewing encourages the unfolding and development of understanding as the researcher progresses from interview to interview. In seeking to satisfy themselves that their understanding is as full as it can be, that is, theoretical saturation within the data, grounded theory interviewers will adapt and change their questioning. They try to strike a balance between directing interviews and not cutting off interesting theoretical leads, relying on pre-formulated questions or loading too many assumptions into their questioning. However, this apparent lack of structure can be anxiety provoking for some researchers who prefer the structure afforded by a semi-structured interview schedule. In our experience, this tension can be managed using a semi-structured format that is 'loose'. The initial research questions arise from the researcher's curiosity, clinical and life experience, and reading. It is highly likely the researcher will have read some relevant literature, particularly in research degree programmes that do require a brief literature review in the research proposal that supports the research aims, despite the grounded theory study requirement to set aside the more formal literature review until later in the process of the analysis. These early research questions can be listed and grouped. There is no requirement to ask all the questions, or to ask them in the same order, with each initial participant. The grounded theory method of constant comparison provides the sounding board on which further questions are developed and other questions dropped, as interviewing and analysis proceed side by side.

In direct contrast, structured interviews require either short, specific responses to questions provided by the interviewer or open responses subsequently categorized by the interviewer. The same questions are asked in the same order to all participants. Whilst this limits what the interviewee can say, and does not actively promote an empathic relationship within the interview process, it has the advantage of quickness and reliability.

Semi-structured interviews maximize rapport between the interviewer and participant. The ordering and phrasing of the questions is less important, as follow-up and probe questions can be used to explore and develop interesting leads. The more natural conversational context provided by the semi-structured interview has the advantage of taking the interviewer into new areas of enquiry not anticipated by the research question and literature review. However, an interview process that privileges rapport makes more demands on the interviewer and could raise anxiety in an unhelpful way. We sometimes find that otherwise accomplished clinical interviewers become tongue-tied during their early research interviews. We see this as part of the process of skills transfer and it emphasizes the need for supervision, practice and pilot work.

In sum, we can see interviews on a continuum, ranging from structured interviews, where interviewers try to maximize control, through semi-structured to unstructured whereby the respondent shares more in the construction of the interview. However we structure our questions, it is important to consider their sequence and flow, much as we would in a clinical interview. For example, we may start with some introductory and orientative remarks, followed by some warm-up questions and the main questions of the interview, which is ended with some cool-off questions, further feedback and the close of the interview. Such pacing pays attention to the comfort of the interviewee.

## Consequences

Much has been written about the practical aspects of interviewing and the analysis of interview material, but less so about the ethical question of whom the interview is for, and what implications that has for sampling and reciprocity in the research relationship. We write about sampling in Chapter 3. Here though, we wish to acknowledge that different interests and purposes can be served through interviewing. It is also helpful to consider how interviewers' and interviewees' intentions and motivations to seek information and opinions, to give of themselves and to enter into a dialogue to explore further and in some depth the implications and consequences of their positioning around topics and experiences can be profound. In psychotherapy based research, acknowledgement of this potential complexity is crucial to establishing some reciprocity in the interviewing relationship, particularly when we ask people to disclose around sensitive and personal topics. Such acknowledgement can be woven into the interview process, discussed before and after the interview and, in our view, should be considered as part of the 'data' for analysis.

Thus we can appreciate how both the interviewer and the interviewee are cultural anthropologists, interested in illuminating understanding of some phenomenon, although their perspectives and intents will be different. They both take turns to be listener and speaker, whereby speaking and listening are equally valued, and the experience of meeting each other will have a provocative impact for both of them.

## CONJOINT INTERVIEWING

The above discussion is based on the assumption that we are interviewing one person at a time. Perhaps we see more clearly the interrelationship between what people say and what we observe in interviews when we interview more than one person at once. Some research studies interview couples, family groups, work teams and so on. In these circumstances we are interviewing people who have pre-existing emotional relationships with each other, that can be described as more or less intense, committed, equal and so on, but perhaps most importantly from our point of view as potential interviewers, their relationship will continue once the interview has ended. We see this illustrated when interviewing conjointly around sensitive topics, such as domestic violence. For example, Liz Bonham's (personal communication) research with heterosexual couples, where the men had behaved violently towards the women in the past, seeks to explore how the men think they decided to stop being violent, how the women think the men took this decision and what helped the men keep to their decision. After such an interview, we might worry if the woman's safety has been compromised, in terms of what they decided to tell the researcher and how they told it.

So, in thinking about a research interview as an intervention into people's lives, if we interview couples, say, how might they position themselves in their interview? Are they more concerned about presenting themselves as a loving united couple? Does one of them see it as an opportunity to 'put one over' on the other, or undermine the other in front of an outsider? Or do they not care much what the interviewer thinks of them as a couple? This might indicate that much can be learned from the interview by watching their interaction as a couple, making some process notes during or after the interview and using these interpretations to help with the analysis of the interview. In addition, we should note that sometimes we find ourselves interviewing someone in the presence of another, either invited or uninvited! For example, researchers who ask children about their experiences in family therapy sessions will often interview children at home, in the presence of a parent (Lobatto, 2002). We need to consider how responding can be both facilitated and constrained under these circumstances. An interview study by Drummond and Mason (1990), exploring the experiences of people living with diabetes, found that often they could not persuade partners to leave the room, so they invited participation from the perspective of 'what it was like to live with a person with diabetes'.

Let us think about these processes further. It could be said that our interviewer's main task is to develop a working alliance with both of them, so that the topic under discussion can be explored as fully as possible. Barry Mason (2003), in his research interviews with heterosexual couples, where the men had been suffering from a chronically painful condition for many years, noted that some of the women partners spoke for the men. The women spoke both about the men's pain and how the men's experience of pain impacted upon their relationship, almost seeming to hold the 'memory' for the couple. Mason's task was to manage the interview process so that he could get a reasonable amount of information and reflections from both partners, without offending the women as informants. As therapists we have a sense of how partners use each other as an audience in a clinical couples interview, and as research interviewers we may find one or both partners tries to draw us into their relationship process, as an ally, mediator and so on. Given our own personal histories, we may find ourselves feeling more sympathetic to one partner. We may be aware of this pull during the interview, or subsequently on reflection with our research supervisor.

If we are concerned that one interviewee in a couples interview might steal the scene, so to speak, we might consider the benefits of combining joint interviewing with individual interviewing, taking advantage of the perceived benefits of both approaches and offering equity to each of the participants (Arksey, 1996). For example, joint interviewing allows us to explore a consensual picture, the different kinds of information and understanding held by the two partners, and allows the partners to fill in each other's memory gaps. Disadvantages could include one person dominating another, mutual distraction or stirring up unhelpful tensions and disagreements. Following up a joint interview with two individual interviews, allows factual data to be cross-checked, gives voice to both participants and throws into relief different perceptions and tensions within the couple. However, we should recognize that combined interviewing places a heavier burden of participation on our respondents, and there is some suggestion that participation rates are lower in these studies, raising questions around the nature of volunteer status for our data (Pahl, 1989). In contrast to this, Gale (1992) reported a research study that used regular conjoint research interviewing to identify significant events during therapy, both during and after couples therapy. The research couples reported that the research interviews, which encouraged recursive self-reflection, were sometimes more therapeutic than the couples therapy itself! In part, this seemed to occur because of the nature of the research relationship, the contextualization and constraints of the research talk, and the procedures used by the research interview to clarify the couples' experiences and understandings.

In summary, the data obtained from individual and conjoint interviews are qualitatively different. The first is more an individualized account of events and opinions, whereas the second is jointly constructed in the presence of an 'outsider' to their relationship. So, although the interviewee and interviewer can be said to co-construct an 'individual' interview, once an interviewer meets a couple, with a prior emotional relationship, they may encounter different social processes, invested with different and possibly more intense meanings, in the process of the interview itself. From the researcher's perspective, conjoint interviewing can be more personally demanding and exhausting, for example, trying to ensure some equality of participation and trying to help manage tension and disagreement during the interview.

## FOCUS GROUPS

Focus groups have come to prominence recently in social research. We consider them here as an interesting variant on conjoint interviewing. As in our discussion of interviewing and observation above, they can be used within both critical realist and social constructionist paradigms. They find their place in psychotherapy research in how they help us understand a phenomenon from the point of view of a group of people, for example, in exploring consistency between scientific explanations and everyday knowledge. They have the potential to raise consciousness and empower participants and have been used extensively to explore service users' views. As an example of this use, Curle and Mitchell (2004) convene a focus group of service users to consult on the development and implementation of clinical psychology training curricula.

Fern (2001) suggests focus groups can be used to clarify decision making processes, and for theory applications, such as the development of theoretical ideas. Developing this distinction, Fern argues that focus groups can be adapted for three research tasks:

1 Exploratory – creating, collecting, identifying, discovering, explaining and generating thoughts, feelings and behaviours, from which the researcher might generate theory through an inductive process.
2 Experiential – the observation of 'natural attitudes' and learned behaviours that we take for granted in our lives, as manifest in shared life experiences, preferences, intentions and behaviours.
3 Clinical – uncovering individual motives, most commonly used in marketing research, where researchers are less interested in whether the ideas are unique or shared.

Focus groups can be used collaboratively, creatively and flexibly. In our experience as research supervisors, we find that focus groups can be used in a number of ways:

■ As the main vehicle for data collection, whereby one or more focus groups are convened to discuss the research question, and then convened again, and perhaps again, to develop thinking further, in an ethno-methodological manner.

- As part of a pilot strategy that helps to clarify and hone the main research question.
- As part of a validation strategy, whereby the researcher takes the research findings to a focus group of research participants (or to a 'similar' group of people) for their views on the validity and applicability of the findings and for further discussion on the future development of the main research question.
- In three-stage action research, where a focus group of interested parties is convened to help shape the research question around a common interest or problem; the participants are then interviewed individually, and then the analysis of the interviews is taken back to the same focus group for further discussion and development.
- Where parallel focus groups have been convened that represent different perspectives within an organization – for example, service users, clinicians and service managers, or different professions within multidisciplinary clinical services – or where the different perspectives are contained within the same focus group – for example, where a multiprofessional team acts as the focus group.

Clearly, there are advantages and disadvantages to convening homogenous and heterogenous groups. For example, more powerful people and views may predominate, too much homogeneity could restrict thinking and too much heterogeneity could be unable to examine what is held in common, or the group might focus on similarity of views rather than difference. Fern (2001) argues that exploratory and clinical focus groups are interested in differences across individuals within the groups, whereas experiential focus groups are interested in sameness within the group. Thus facilitating focus groups is a skilled task, that draws heavily on clinical experiences of understanding and managing group processes. As such, it is suited to the needs and skills of psychotherapist researchers.

Focus groups are efficient. They enable research on those topics that relate to group norms, to the meanings that might underpin those norms and the group processes whereby those meanings are co-constructed. In particular, focus groups enjoy an advantage where group norms may be hidden or countercultural. They allow a number of views to be collected simultaneously; they are enjoyable, quick and cheap to run; and they provide opportunities for ice-breaking and stimulating discussion around taboo subjects and for participation for people who may not otherwise take part in social research.

Focus group discussion usually lasts between one and two hours, in which time about six to ten main questions can be addressed. In our experience, groups of about six to eight participants are easier to manage, whereby all participants can be encouraged to speak and explore differences with a sense of safety. The enlivening nature of group discussion can sometimes lead to the researcher being carried away with enthusiasm, losing sight of their need to warrant their findings in other ways! Wherever possible, we suggest the researcher is joined by a second researcher, often a colleague or another student on the same course. A lone researcher faces the choice of whether they facilitate the group, or observe the group and manage the discussion task set by the researcher whilst he or she takes notes. A second researcher can run the group, leaving the first researcher freer to observe and take notes during the discussion. As therapists we are all well used to facilitating workshops and have often participated in them ourselves as learners. Adapting our tried and tested workshop formats with their focus on experiential learning through discussion provides the expertise we need.

Focus groups are often audio recorded for subsequent transcription and analysis. Obviously, it can be harder to discern who is speaking from the audio-tape. If possible, holding the discussion in a therapy suite that has video-recording facilities available is preferable. The focus group discussion will have been directed and focused during the time available, and the facilitator will have jotted key points of the discussion on flip-chart paper as the discussion evolved. This leaves the researcher with three kinds of data: the direct output of the group; the audio/video recording; and process observation notes made during the group. Data analysis and interpretation can use many of the qualitative methods, such as, theme analysis, interpretative phenomenological analysis, and discourse analysis. Interactional analyses have not been much used to date, perhaps reflecting the development of focus groups within market research. The context of the groups will influence the analytic method chosen, as will the researcher's understanding of theories of group processes.

Despite the current popularity of focus groups, there is not much critical literature available to guide the researcher. Caution needs to be exercised in assuming that the conclusions are warranted. For example, the focus group is exploring collective views, not individual views, so generalization of findings at best, is to theory, rather than to other individuals or populations. The range of views held within the group may be revealed, but not necessarily the depth of views. Finally, they may not represent a consensus view, as hoped, but they might reveal splits in opinions or recurring themes and concerns.

## THE DELPHI METHOD

The Delphi method is included in our discussion of methods of 'conjoint interviewing' as an example of structured and iterative survey work. The method rests in the philosophical assumption that 'n heads are better than one' (Dalkey, 1972). The procedure samples the opinions of a group of knowledgeable persons in an attempt to seek consensus on complex topics, such as, the essential elements of the supervisory process or the comparison of the main features of rival schools of psychotherapy, or to plan policy issues for a discipline or field of practice, such as working with domestic violence. The aim is more with the potential application of useful knowledge than concerns about the status of truth. Research participants are invited to offer their views anonymously. The researcher gathers feedback from the panel of participants, and then offers this collected feedback to the panel, who may revise their views if they so wish upon reading the views of the other participants. Arguably, this method reduces pressure for group consensus from dominant persons whilst preserving the benefits of group dialogue. The researcher structures the process of group communication and thus is not involved in the expense of convening a face-to-face meeting of knowledgeable persons (Stone Fish and Busby, 1996).

The Delphi method has not been widely used amongst psychotherapy researchers, but we think it has untapped potential for exploring theoretical and practice dilemmas. For example, Liz Burns (2003, unpublished PhD thesis) was interested in the extent to which senior family therapists used aspects of their own experience in their therapeutic work and, in particular, how they incorporated their reading of novels, poetry and plays into their practice.

Delphi panellists are chosen for their expertise, rather than in a random or adventitious way. Data collection is by questionnaire, with stability of response usually achieved within two to three rounds (Linstone and Turoff, 1975). Initially, the participants are invited to write as much as they wish about the topic under study. The researcher then pools the information, looking for agreement and disagreement within the panel responses. Themes or categories are developed, using the participants' language. These pooled responses are then sent out to the panel, so they can re-evaluate their answers based on the group feedback. Panellists are often asked to rate the pooled items, so the data may be subject to analysis of group agreement, using medians and interquartile ranges. There are some disadvantages to this method of seeking consensus. For example, diversity is minimized, the initial categories may be too broad and after two to three rounds there may be a regression to the mean in responding.

As an example, White and Russell (1995) used the Delphi method to identify variables thought to be important to the outcome of couple and family therapy supervision. They wanted to collect empirical data where none existed. Their longer term aim was to develop a model of supervision, and facilitate research into the process of couple and family therapy supervision. They selected a Delphi panel from the AAMFT list of approved supervisors. Sixty-one panellists completed both rounds of the study. The panel generated 771 variables thought to be important to supervisory outcome. In the second round, the panel rated 398 of these variables as very important. These variables were then collapsed into five categories, consisting of 37 conceptual clusters: supervisor variables; supervisee variables; supervisor–supervisee relationship variables; supervisory interaction variables; and contextual variables.

## INTERPERSONAL PROCESS RECALL

We introduce the method of interpersonal process recall here as it is a very structured form of in-depth interviewing and can be used with single and multiple respondents. Elliott (1986) has pioneered work on enlisting clients, therapists and observers as collaborators in analysing their own significant therapy events. The focus of the interview is to learn as much as possible about the significant events and about the reasons for the differences among the perspectives. In fact it was Elliott's research that first indicated how discrepant the three points of view could be! Significant

events are portions of therapy sessions, usually a few minutes long, identified as being most helpful or important. These events are assumed to
illuminate the process of change in psychotherapy. The study of significant
events is a sampling strategy – an attempt to look for concentrated
moments of therapeutic action. The therapy session is either audio-taped or
video-taped. Immediately afterwards, research participants are asked to
identify any helpful events using the HAT questionnaire (see below) and,
with tape-assisted recall, to identify where in the session the helpful
event(s) took place. Elliott argues that careful, open-ended description of
these events illuminates therapeutic change processes, within a specific
context, and thereby contributes to improvements in the practice of
psychotherapy.

## Comprehensive process analysis

CPA (Comprehensive Process Analysis) (Elliott, 1989) was developed to
analyse both individual helpful events and themes across events. The
CPA method focuses on four areas of understanding:

1 Expanding the key or peak responses in the event, such as exploring the
   implied meanings carried within a response.
2 The *context* out of which the event arises, and that gives it meaning, such
   as what had been happening before or after the event, the nature of
   the therapeutic alliance, background features of client and therapist, the
   client's preferred ways of coping, cultural attunement of the therapy and
   so on.
3 The important *features* of the event itself, such as therapist action, interpretation and style, and client expression of thoughts and feelings.
4 The *impacts* of the event, such as understanding, anticipated changes,
   changes in mood and so on.

The CPA method uses the Helpful Aspects of Therapy Questionnaire (HAT)
(Llewelyn *et al.*, 1988). Immediately after the psychotherapy session, the
client and therapist complete the HAT questionnaire in which they identify
one or more helpful (or unhelpful) events in the preceding session. They
write a brief open-ended description of the event(s) and use the tape recording to identify where the event took place. They agree the beginning and
end of the sequence, and then the researcher helps them deconstruct the
event using the CPA method.

However, it is possible to conduct smaller-scale studies in which only the
responses to the HAT are analysed. The descriptions of the helpful (and/or
unhelpful) events can be rated on a five-point scale for their overall helpfulness. Again using five-point scales, each event can be rated in terms of its
contribution to the following nine areas:

1 Personal insight
2 Problem clarification
3 Problem solution
4 Understanding about others

5 Increase in understanding
6 Reassurance
7 Sense of relief
8 Involvement in the therapy
9 Personal contact with the therapist.

In addition, the participants can describe in what ways the session was helpful *overall* and then rate the session *overall* for its helpfulness. Using five-point scales, the therapy session can be rated overall in terms of its contribution to the nine areas listed above. The open-ended descriptions of both the helpful events and the sessions can be theme or content analysed. We have used the HAT to review the overall helpfulness of therapy itself at the close of the therapeutic work. It has also been developed to explore the helpful aspects of supervision, where supervisors and supervisees can identify helpful events in supervision, in supervision sessions and across a range of supervision meetings.

Both of us supervised the research of Marc van Roosmalen (2001). He was interested in the development of the therapeutic alliance and what factors sustained it over the course of therapy with families seeking support from a Tier Three intervention service. The families were raising children, one or more of whom was subject to social services childcare proceedings. He used the method of interpersonal process recall to interview parents and children separately, after the first therapy session, and then after each second session. His analysis of the identified helpful events indicated that the therapeutic alliance was strengthened by an approach that took into account the developmental needs of the children and was child-centred; the alliance with the parents was strengthened by an approach that helped the parents shift their understanding of the problem from a blame focus on the child to a more contextual understanding of causation. The therapeutic alliance was also strengthened by all family members' perception of the therapist as genuinely interested in all their points of view and experiences in a way that enhanced their sense of participation in the therapeutic work. His work provides us with an example of do-able research, conducted in a way that maximizes collaborative enquiry and generates findings of use to other practitioners.

## QUESTIONNAIRE DESIGN

Some research questions require a more controlled and standardized situation to reduce sources of variance in responding. The researcher might choose to design a short questionnaire as a postal or telephone survey, or as the basis of a structured interview, in which each question is asked in turn, in the same manner for all participants. Often with such structured interviewing, the researcher is more interested in the direct responses to the questions, and the analysis proceeds on that basis, usually categorizing and counting responses.

Questionnaires need to be efficient and usable. The respondent needs to have enough information about the study to be able to answer the questions. The questionnaire needs to be personalized and attractive to reduce non-response. Flash cards and other pictorial means can be used to prompt responses, and can be particularly helpful when interviewing younger children. Items in structured interviews do not need to be as brief, nor the response categories as limited as for telephone surveys.

There are some general rules for writing questionnaire questions that we summarize here:

1  Questions should be short, clear and focused. Avoid too many open-ended questions, vague or complex questions, double-barrelled and leading questions; if a question can be misinterpreted, it will be!
2  When asking multiple choice questions, be sure they are mutually exclusive. Response alternatives are best contained in the question, with ranking questions limited to three to four items.
3  When asking people to recall past events, provide a temporal frame. For example, how many times in the past six months did you see your counsellor? Try to avoid asking for information on probabilities and proportions.
4  When using scaling questions, provide meaningful 'anchors'.
5  Ease of coding for numeric responses is important. For example, categories (nominal/ordinal; or none, 1–10, 11–20, 21–30+) or scales (interval/ratio). Verbal responses can be coded numerically, such as regularly, often, seldom, never, or always, often, sometimes, seldom, never.
6  In both survey questionnaires and structured interviews, group the questions together by content and place related items together.
7  Put the questions that are directly related to the survey objectives first, with the most problematic or sensitive questions at the end of each section. Finish the questionnaire with demographic items.
8  Phone surveys are generally shorter with fewer categories used.
9  Always remember the survey's purpose. If in doubt about a question, do not use it.

Non-response to questionnaires is not a problem if the non-respondents do not differ from the respondents in terms of the survey variables. However, the lower the response rate, the more likely it is there is a difference. Non-response is lower when the perceived cost of completion is low and the benefit is high. Always check for systematic non-response. Follow-up mailings can sometimes help in improving response rates, but note the possibility of differential responding between those who reply earlier and those who reply later. Brief questionnaires and telephone surveys are often used by psychotherapists when seeking client and referrer feedback. Viljoen and Wolpert (2002), writing from the context of child and adolescent mental health services, suggest a number of ways for improving return rates from postal outcome questionnaires, such as, anonymity, respondent friendly (and brief!) designs, monetary incentives, handing out question-naires personally, using a cover letter that includes an appeal, stamped addressed envelopes for return, colour of the questionnaire and prior notice.

## THE RELATIONSHIP BETWEEN OBSERVATION AND INTERVIEWING AS RESEARCH ACTIVITIES

In our experience, the two data-gathering methods of observation and interviewing invariably go together. For example, during observation, people usually talk. During an interview, we also observe and, arguably, we use the non-verbal data both explicitly and implicitly in our understanding and interpretation of the data. We see this process at work most clearly in the transcription of our interviews, or subsequent editing of our interviews. If our interview audio tapes have been transcribed by someone else who was not present during the interview, the task of editing is crucial. We may edit back in long pauses and hesitations in the talk, or expressions of effect, like laughter and tearfulness, or discrepancies between what people are saying and what they appear to be feeling, or our experiences of discomfort at certain points in the interview, and so on. The interview transcript, in our view, can never be an accurate reflection of the interview itself. For us, it is axiomatic: that in understanding an interview situation we appreciate that more than one point of view is involved. It was Goffman (1959) who said: 'Many crucial facts lie beyond the time and place of interaction, or lie concealed within it.'

Thus we proceed with caution when relying exclusively on interviews as a source of data. In Chapter 10 we talk about the use of triangulated methodologies as a means of enhancing the trustworthiness of our study findings, for example, combining interview data with observational data. What we wish to discuss here is the potential for using our approach to interpretative observational analysis whilst doing an interview study, in order to harness the benefits of observational approaches.

Certain dilemmas can arise when we interrelate what we hear with what we see during an interview. For example, we may have recorded our interview on audio-tape, and then recorded our responses to the interview afterwards in our research journal, such as our sense of how we got on with our interviewee, whether we agreed or disagreed with what they were saying and whether we were confused or worried by apparent discrepancies between what they were saying and their accompanying non-verbal behaviour. Such reflections are crucial to our understanding of our own interpretative activity during the interviews, how that might have influenced the course of the interview and how our inferences may then impact within the data analysis and subsequent write-up. This is known as self-reflexivity in the clinical and research literature and as such is encouraged but, in our view, with little written about how we might approach it, especially in research journal articles. For us, it is crucial to our understanding of the interview situation that we appreciate that more than one perspective is involved.

As clinical researchers we have to make decisions about what to pay attention to, during and after interviews, and how we might interpret this. The work of the MRI theorists on analogue and digital communication can help us here (Watzlawick et al., 1967). We have all probably experienced ourselves and others talking and behaving in apparently contradictory ways, such as the person who tells you they are not angry through clenched teeth, while tensing their fist and slitting their eyes. Carrying on with our example above, our interview analysis may rely on grounded methods, discursive methods, or a combination of both. Whatever method of analysis we choose, the interpretative activity based on our observations of what people are saying during an interview, and the way in which we experience them saying it, needs to be considered within the following four frameworks:

1  What is the person communicating, both verbally and non-verbally?
2  How am I responding to them, both verbally and non-verbally?
3  What do I think is going on between us at this point?
4  What are the contextual influences within and outwith the interview?

Our chosen method of interview data analysis might lead us to pay attention to one of these frameworks more than another. For example, a grounded analysis would focus more on framework 1, while a discursive analysis might focus more on framework 3. For us, a full interpretative observational analysis study will consider all four frameworks equally, whatever our main analytic approach.

Another dilemma concerns whether we accept at 'face value' what people say in an interview, or whether we think we have to 'interpret', theoretically speaking, what we hear. A number of factors would tend to lean us more in one direction than the other:

- Our own epistemological positioning, such as a more constructivist, critical realist or a social constructionist view of talk, perception, interaction and context, that might lead us to assume ideas expressed in interaction can be relatively stable, or not.
- Our preferred theoretical frameworks, such as psychodynamic, which might lead us to believe that people speak from intrapsychically defended positions, both interviewers and interviewees (Hollway and Jefferson, 2000).
- Our understanding of our relative roles and expectations of each other during the interview and our relative power positions, for example, a therapist interviewing a client, a junior doctor interviewing a consultant and so on. We would suggest that the use of an interpretative observational analysis framework helps us address and resolve the dilemmas between latent and manifest content within interviews.
- How we understand the place and function of non-verbal interaction during the interview, and what importance we place on congruence between verbal and non-verbal forms of communication.

In relation to Hollway and Jefferson's point, raised above, our approach to interpretative observational analysis is to annotate our interview transcripts. Immediately after the interview, take further notes on the context for the interviewer and the participant, for example, where the interview took place and how that might affect the process, the anxieties and vested interests held. Take notes from the perspective of the interviewer and the participant on what ideas might have been developed, suppressed and/or linked during the interview. In particular, identify inconsistencies and puzzling links, threats to safety and how they were resolved, and the use of metaphors and other cultural symbols. Identify larger discourses at play in the interview text. These analytical process notes can be used to both contextualize the interview and to complement subsequent qualitative analysis. They can be subjected to reflexive self analysis to help identify our own positioning in relation to the context, topic and participation within the interview.

## PARTICIPANT OBSERVATION AND DEPTH INTERVIEWING: SIMILARITIES AND DIFFERENCES

In this section we consider the question often asked by research students: how do I know when to use participative observational methods or an in-depth approach to interviewing? For us, both methods of enquiry offer rich and detailed approaches to social behaviour, but the crux of the answer lies in the formulation of the research question. Approaches to participant observation proceed inductively, on the basis that understandings of social interactions cannot be ascertained only by asking individuals questions about their behaviour. On the other hand, in-depth interviewing procedures are deductive, based on the premise that we cannot directly observe the development of personal accounts, belief systems and narratives. Thus, if we start our enquiry with a question informed by previous research or theory, we can proceed quite quickly to in-depth interviewing as our main strategy for gathering data. Conversely, the observational approach is indicated when we start with a strategic interest in a particular research site, such as a recurring clinical observation. It may be the case that there is not a pre-existing empirical or theoretical literature on which we might draw.

Both approaches can be used in a culturally sensitive way and offer reflexivity of approach, whereby researchers can draw out cultural descriptions from others while providing cultural descriptions of themselves as researchers. So-called hidden dimensions of culture can be sought by using supplemental questions and observations. It is often in our interpretation of how these methods should be used that we find ethnocentrism. In our experience, it is the researcher's ability to perceive and conceptualize, grounding the literature, the data and the cultural context in a mutually influential way, that makes for a culturally nuanced study.

For example, AV's interest in patterning in family behaviour led her to approach family groups to seek permission to make naturalistic observations in people's own homes. Her approach was based on the assumption that observation was needed to capture the everyday flux of family life. Interestingly, family therapists, who talk to family members in therapists' offices, assume they will both observe social interactions amongst family members whilst talking with them about the felt quality of family life in an ecologically valid way.

In developing a research strategy, the use of in-depth interviewing or participant observation implies different types and degrees of preparation. For example, interviewing requires piloting to develop both the interview schedule and to help with sample selection. This may include early theoretical analysis, based on existing work in the field. Meanwhile, the participant observer can enter the field once the research site has been negotiated. It is often the case that research questions develop and are further refined as the observational activity progresses. As we saw in Chapter 8, in the description of the possible social roles of the participant observer, the observer does not rely only on watching and hearing, but actively engages at times in listening within conversational encounters. The difference being, of course, that these conversational opportunities are taking place in the day-to-day activities of the research participants and do not follow a pre-prepared interview format set by the observer.

Preparation assumes that the researcher considers both intra-cultural and inter-cultural issues, such as gender, class and ethnicity, when planning a study and seeking research participation. It may be that such issues form part of the research question, and early pilot work may seek to compare and contrast findings across small theoretically derived sample groups. In our experience, consideration of intra-cultural and inter-cultural issues means that we need to identify how our research aims sit within different community groups and how our interests may complement their interests, or not, as the case may be! When working cross-culturally, early preparation often means extensive consultation with community leaders, seeking their interest and approval and explaining how our research may be of benefit to the community (Turner, 2000). Such a commitment often leads to collaborative research designs, where culture can be seen as a map, but sensitivity is maintained to intra-group differences. The phenomenological focus brought by both in-depth interviewing and participant observation approaches helps maintain a balance between shared and distinct characteristics and intra-group variation.

Another question often asked, is whether and to what extent an interview should be structured. Interviews are usually structured along a continuum from unstructured through semi-structured to structured. We shall not consider structured interviews here, as the structured format, of asking the same questions to each participant in the same order, does not have the in-built flexibility to help refine the research question as part of the method of enquiry. Instead, we shall consider unstructured and semi-structured interview formats, which challenge the interviewer to explore and develop ideas as they unfold during an interview encounter. Clearly, experience and pilot work help to build the interviewer's confidence that they are able to get the most out of an interview, but still it remains a conceptual and social challenge to carry out an interview that progresses research practice and thinking. Arguably, counsellors and psychotherapists bring with them a wealth of clinical experience wherein they use the clinical interview as the medium for the development of the therapeutic relationship and thus the vehicle for change. The ethical question arises as to the differences and similarities within research and clinical interviews that we need to keep in mind. Researchers will probably acknowledge that research interviews are short and contractual and do not occur within an ongoing supportive relationship found in clinical interviewing. Thus there have to be limits on what it is permissible to pursue as a justifiable research lead, that does not lead us to stray into a quasi-therapeutic interview. Although it could be argued many clinically driven research questions can lead to an interviewing style that is therapeutic, and possibly of personal benefit to the interviewee, our research participants are not usually in a position to give *informed* consent, in that we need to undergo an experience to know what it is we are consenting to!

On the other hand, Gale (1992) discusses when research interviews can be more therapeutic than therapy interviews. In conducting research that examined a couple's and therapist's perceptions of meaningful moments in therapy using the interpersonal process recall methodology (Elliott, 1986), the couple reported the research interviews to be more helpful than the therapy itself. This seemed to be because the IPR method itself involved the use of clarifying procedures by the researcher, the nature of the relationship with the researcher, and the context of the 'research talk'. The nature of the IPR method is such that it invites people to be self-reflexive and is recursive in nature. The researcher's need to clarify the couple's understanding and experience led to the use of analogy, which the couple themselves elaborated. This seemed to lead to a retelling of their experience that allowed new meaning and punctuations to emerge, or as the researcher's said, 'the unsaid of the therapy session could be explored and rewritten through the collaborative effort of developing new descriptions'. The researcher found that the couple could laugh at their own interactions during the IPR procedure and both acknowledged new responsibilities and appreciations for behaviour. The researcher speculated that the collaborative and reciprocal nature of the research enquiry, combined with the 'psychological distance' involved in reviewing taped interaction as part of the IPR method, created a context for learning and interpersonal growth.

Interviews can be thought of as theoretical projects. As researchers we need to develop interview questions and ways of asking them that antici-pate and uncover a range of contexts within which the research question has relevance. Whether we think interviews are designed to discover par-ticipants' ways of thinking about the social world (such as might be found within a constructivist frame of reference, perhaps using the IPA as a method of analysis) or that meanings are co-constructed in interviews (such as might be found with a social constructionist approach, perhaps using a discourse analysis), we need to consider the limitations of talk and text and the problems of self-report data. Interview studies make the assumption that key aspects of our social experiences and practices can be captured with dialogue, but as Hollway and Jefferson (2000) put it, 'people are not their own best explainers'. They take the view that our largely unconscious ways of coping with external threats to our well-being and safety go a long way towards understanding who we are. People may engage in a number of strategies designed to put their 'best foot forward', ranging from impression management through to answering questions we did not ask them, under-pinned by the demand characteristics of the interview and interviewees' attempts to second guess the 'real' intentions of the researcher (Orne, 1962; Rosenhan, 1973; Rosenthal, 1976). Methodologically speaking, we need to question whether reliance on the interview as the main method of data gathering presupposes the existence of the articulate and rational social actor. Triangulation strategies, discussed elsewhere in the text, offer one way round some of the above dilemmas. Alternatively, analytical process notes taken immediately after the interview (as discussed above) can inform our self-reflexive analysis.

In order to carry out an exploratory participant observation study, we need to gain access to a research site or research group. Problems of access and sampling have been discussed elsewhere (see Chapters 3 and 8), but suffice to say here, a model of gaining access is important, in both mapping and understanding any organizational opportunities and barriers to the research site. Such a modelling process helps predict the sampling strategy, and the effects of early sampling upon the developing nature of the research question. The researcher is engaged in a continuous and iterative process of observing, recording, analysing, categorizing and linking. The participant observer has to contend with some major challenges to validity, such as problems of sampling, researcher bias, reactivity and changes in both the observer and observed over time (Vetere and Gale, 1987). The task of the therapeutically trained research observer is to try to note the small and apparently trivial, without too much a priori clinical theorizing driving the research question at this stage. So, as we noted above with the dilemma of doing both clinical and research interviews, clinicians are likely to make good observers, in that they can pay attention to detail and have good memory for sequential events, but are likely to suffer from thinking they have seen this before.

Whether we choose the methods of observation or in-depth interviewing, life as a field researcher is enjoyable, anxiety provoking and potentially exhausting. Our clinical training and experiences with professional supervision make it likely that we have developed an approach to working under such conditions. So, for us, ongoing research supervision is essential, both to develop our reflexivity in relation to our research enquiry and to maintain some balance between our personal and professional lives. The semi-structured in-depth interview is most like a clinical interview, in that self-disclosure is encouraged and made possible. It provides an opportunity for the interviewee to reflect on their usual social interactions, meanings and motives. As a parallel process, the researcher is encouraged to reflect on the impact of the interview process on them and on their subsequent thinking, in a research diary, in supervision and so on, and used as part of a grounded and reflective analysis. The grounded theory method of constant comparison allows the significance of any one interview to be compared with another, such that links and hypotheses can be developed until theoretical saturation is reached. By way of contrast, the participant observer makes real time observations, within the flow of everyday social exchanges. The observer is in a position to watch events and relationships as they develop over time. The observational role is time consuming, with the potential for moving between the social roles of the participant observer (see Chapter 8) and for varying the degree to which they hold an 'outsider' perspective.

Whether we have chosen to conduct in-depth interviews or observations, we need to make decisions about how we leave the field and withdraw from our relationships with our research participants. Arguably, this is easier with a research study organized around a series of interviews with different people, rather than with a study which seeks to re-interview the same respondents, or where we have spent time in proximity with people as part of an observational study, where our research relationships might be enduring and more meaningful, emotionally speaking. Thus it could be said the design of a one-off semi-structured interview carries less burden for the research participant. This is because of its attention to the stages of opening the interview, conducting the interview and closing the interview, within an ethical framework which allows participants to withdraw from the interview at any time and which seeks to safety net any emotional consequences of participating in an interview. However, this might not be so. An interview on a sensitive topic might evoke predictable and unpredictable responses, including those that are relatively unprocessed, emotionally speaking. This can be a risk for both the research interviewer and the research interviewee, and raises for us the interesting and complex question of how and in what ways a research interview is the same as, and different from, a clinical interview.

As clinicians we are used to seeking informed consent to therapy procedures as an ongoing process of discovery, where pacing can be adjusted to suit the needs of our client groups. This may not be so practicable in one-off in-depth interviews, which by their very nature seek some degree of genuine engagement with the topic on behalf of both parties to the research. Thus careful attention needs to be given to how we close interviews and withdraw from the observational field. Our clinical experience can be enormously helpful here: preparation and procedures for ending are built in from the start; negotiation of any continuing contact is governed by our respective codes of conduct; helpful contacts for dealing with the effects of the research are provided; and summaries of the research findings are made available at the end of the research. All of these practices explicitly acknowledge the impact of the research intervention on people's lives.

The final difference between the two methodologies we wish to address here concerns the analyses of the data. The analysis of observational data is often focused on interactional patterns within the group under observation. Interactions, however defined, can form the basic unit of analysis. The ongoing and complementary nature of data collection and analysis within an observational study promotes the generation of hypotheses and linkages between hypotheses in a manner that mimics clinical observation and formulation, particularly in areas of working that are not rich in clinical theorizing. On the other hand, the analysis of in-depth interview material tends to focus on individual characteristics, such as attributions of meaning, the use of rhetorical strategies and larger narratives or biographies. The analyses of group based in-depth interviews, such as with couples, families and peer groups, are in their infancy. Apart from the structured methods of focus groups, which arguably do not capture 'depth' of meaning so readily, we need to do further work on refining our analytic methods. However, in-depth interviews provide us with a unique opportunity to examine how wider social changes are perceived and understood and to what extent people think they have a part to play in influencing such processes. It is here that we see another direct parallel with clinical work, in that clinical interviews will often focus on wider social processes that may be said to have some direct bearing on how we see ourselves, ourselves in relation to others, and on our sense of well-being.

So, in summary, we can see that interviewing and observation can be alternative choices, depending on how the research question is theorized, or they can be used in a complementary manner. For example, observational work can pilot and ground a research question within a phenomenon of substance, which can then be further explored in terms of its meaning to participants using in-depth interviews. Alternatively, exploration of the meanings attributed to an event, say, can be complemented by observation of that same event, for example, a cultural or family ritual. This could form part of a triangulated approach to exploration and understanding of human social processes.

## KEY REFERENCE

Fern, E. (2001) *Advanced Focus Group Research*. London: Sage.

# 10  APPROACHES TO VALIDITY

## CHAPTER OVERVIEW

This chapter explores some approaches to establishing the validity and social utility of research findings, in observational studies, quantitative and qualitative studies, including case studies, and in mixed methods studies. The approaches discussed here rely heavily on the involvement of research participants, independent scrutiny from colleagues and transparent processes of data collection and data processing. We argue that if research activity is to embrace principles of collaboration, to encourage the appreciation of clinical experience in research design and to promote reflection, it needs to speak to our needs as clinical practitioners, both as doers of research and consumers of research. This chapter appears at the end of the book because it assumes familiarity with a range of research designs and methods of data collection, discussed in earlier chapters, all of which need to incorporate validity strategies into the design early on. An appreciation of the different validity strategies available, and ideas of how to combine them according to the needs of the research study, will be best achieved once the earlier chapters have been read.

## PUBLISHABILITY GUIDELINES IN QUANTITATIVE AND QUALITATIVE RESEARCH

Validity is a somewhat contested term in the field of qualitative and mixed methods enquiry, despite its long tradition of use in quantitative studies. We take the view that thoughtful and reflexive research builds in approaches to the validity, or trustworthiness (Riessman, 1993), of the findings from the start of the study through to the final write-up. Involving our research participants and our colleagues in the design and scrutiny of our study and in the findings contributes to an open and collaborative stance that emphasizes the importance of experience and clinical practice. Equally, if we seek such collaboration and ask people to give of their time, we need ways of ensuring the practical and social utility of our research work and grounding the research in do-able designs. Thus validity is one of the golden threads that can be tugged at any stage of the research to show how the research process can generate relevant results for theory and practice.

Methods of reliability, validity and replicability support quantitative research, while validity and self-reflexivity support qualitative research. In this chapter, we give an overview of the different approaches to validity that promote our practice as clinical researchers. We shall begin with some discussion of what the quantitative and qualitative paradigms have in common and then draw out some of the differences in their approaches to validity.

The work of Elliott and colleagues (1999) is helpful. They have tried to summarize their understanding of the evolving guidelines for the publishability of qualitative research studies in the social science and clinical practitioner disciplines. They do this in the context of what both quantitative and qualitative paradigms hold in common, and on the assumption that eligibility for publication of research findings is a testament to the social utility of the research. This approach is helpful in that it promotes an attitude of cooperation amongst researchers from different traditions. It also promotes a mixed research economy, something that we strongly favour for clinician researchers, who often find themselves asking complex questions in a very preliminary way.

The publishability guidelines common to both quantitatively and qualitatively informed research approaches include:

- An explicit scientific context and purpose. The research report clearly states the aims and objectives of the study and how the study fits with existing research and theorizing on the topic.

- The use of appropriate methods of enquiry and analysis for the research questions investigated.
- Respect for the research participants and recognition that research is an intervention into people's lives, enshrined in ethical research conduct, such as informed consent for participation, procedures for protecting anonymity, arrangements for the welfare of participants and social responsibility around presentation of the findings.
- Specification of the methods used: reporting on all sampling strategies and procedures used to collect data, including the development of questionnaire or interview protocols, early pilot work; and reporting on the methods used to collect and collate data and all attempts to analyse the data. Such specificity informs researchers who wish to replicate the study or to judge for themselves how well the study was conducted.
- Appropriate discussion of the findings, presented in tentative form, in terms of how the findings sit within the extant literature and their application to current theory and practice, with a critique of the strengths and weaknesses of the study.
- Clarity of presentation of the research. The paper is clearly written and well organized, technical terms are defined, all of which helps the reader find their way about.
- An acknowledged contribution to the development of theory and practice in that area of study.

The publishability guidelines more common to the qualitative approaches, according to Elliott and his colleagues, include:

- Owning one's own perspective and position in relation to the research. Authors identify and make clear their own theoretical orientations, values, biases and assumptions in relation to the research enquiry and how they play in role in the authors' developing analysis and understanding. Such disclosure helps readers to judge for themselves how authors have developed their understandings and to consider possible alternative understandings.
- Situating the sample of participants so that readers are clear about the social and personal contexts of the research participants. This helps readers judge how the findings might be applicable to their practice.
- Grounding the main findings in examples – the audit trail. Detailed examples of the data illustrate both the process of analysis and the development of understandings that allows the reader to examine the fit between the data and the authors' interpretation and to entertain possible alternative interpretations.
- Providing 'credibility' checks for the categories, themes, discourses and accounts produced in the study, using a variety of strategies, such as independent audit, participant checks, comparing multiple perspectives, triangulation strategies and so on.
- The coherence of the data. The arguments and the findings need to be presented in a way that preserves subtleties in the data and allows the reader to appreciate the structure of the data, such as data-based narratives/stories, conversational strategies, thematic frameworks and so on.

- Accomplishing general versus specific research tasks: did the research intend to explore general phenomena or specific phenomena within a case study approach? Are the conclusions and their limitations relevant to the purpose of the study?
- Resonating with the readers, such that the research speaks to the reader's own experiences and practice in a way that clarifies and/or amplifies their own understandings.

## INTERNAL AND EXTERNAL VALIDITY

Cook and Campbell's (1979) definitions of internal and external validity provide a useful set of guidelines for the quantitative clinician researcher. External validity refers to the extent to which the research findings have relevance to real world settings. For example, if we are reading an outcome study of the usefulness of individual psychodynamic psychotherapy, we would want to know to what extent the study findings could translate to our working context as NHS clinicians. So, was the therapy carried out by NHS therapists, in NHS settings, with real NHS users, who represent a range of walks of life, with a range of symptom severity, rather than being carried out by specially trained and well resourced research therapists, in a specialist university setting, with carefully screened research participants? External validity can also be described as ecological validity.

Internal validity, on the other hand, refers to the set of design rules and procedures the study needs to follow to ensure reliability and replicability, underpinned by validity. For example, if we were comparing two forms of family therapy in an outcome study, we would ask questions like: are the participants matched across the two groups and compared with an ethical waiting list control group? Are the methods of family therapy to be compared subject to process checks to see if the therapists are doing what they are supposed to be doing? Are relevant therapist factors known to contribute to different outcomes controlled for within the design? Are pre and post measures of change used, across different perspectives and different response modes? Are the methods of analysis appropriate for the data collected? Is a follow-up period built into the study? If any of these design rules is breached it limits our confidence in the findings and their generalization to practice.

## APPROACHES TO VALIDITY IN OBSERVATIONAL STUDIES

As we have seen in Chapter 8, the use of observation in psychotherapy research can be flexible and creative, as the main source of data, or as part of a mixed methods study approach. The observational process can move along a continuum of a more socially active role for the observer to a more passive role; it can be more or less influenced by a priori theorizing; the data collected can be more or less structured; and the analysis of the data can range from a more constructionist process to a more representational process. The levels of observation and analysis can range from micro processes, such as understanding segments of behaviours or non-verbal movements, to individual behavioural actions, to interactional episodes or sequences of behaviour, to wider macro level processes, such as inter-personal games, and the enactment of roles and 'scripts'. Such variety in observational approaches and types of data presents particular challenges to validity, many of which have been discussed in detail in Chapter 8.

The key issues in observational research are reliability, standardization, sampling and validity. Reliability is a criterion in structured observation that involves coding and measurement. The measures involved need to be reliable and consistent in their use over time, in different contexts and with different observers/raters. Standardization of the coding or rating schemes used in observational studies presumes they have established a basis for making statements about differences. For example, the Camberwell Family Interview (Leff and Vaughn, 1985) purports to measure expressed emotion and show differences in high versus low levels of expressed emotion amongst family members and across diagnostic groups. The sampling strategy needs to be specified, such as: in what contexts and settings did the observation take place, who was present, what were they doing, what 'moods' were sampled, how long did the observation last and at what time of day? The key issues for validity in observational research can be summarized as:

- Face validity – are we measuring/recording/describing what we wish to measure, and does it make sense, logically and theoretically?
- Ecological validity – are we observing the behaviour in its ecologically valid context, such as sibling behaviour at home, or children at play in the schoolyard? Or have we transposed the activity to a more structured environment, such as our clinical base, where we observe carer–child activity through a one-way screen?
- Criterion or external validity – in the study of expressed emotion, how do our observations of parent–adolescent interaction predict future relapse, or risk of relapse?
- Construct validity – does expressed emotion exist as a measurable construct?
- Concurrent validity – how do our observations of expressed emotion correlate with, or agree with, other measures and with accepted indica-tors of expressed emotion, such as relapse, hospitalization and so on?

Our approach to observation, as an active, interpretative activity, involves us in an iterative process of selection, analysis and synthesis. We recognize the multilayered nature of communication and the weave of verbal and non-verbal behaviours over time, including our own, our participants and possible changes for us all over time. Establishing validity can involve seeking corroborating accounts from our participants and other observers; and/or seeking shared accounts that use local and cultural discourses to inform understanding; and/or seeking to replicate our observations with similar scenarios. We describe the contexts of observation carefully, pro-ducing rich accounts and noting patterns in behaviour, process and predictability, often using our clinical experience to inform us. We keep research diaries and reflect on validity and selectivity during and after our observations and during research supervision.

## APPROACHES TO VALIDITY IN QUALITATIVE STUDIES

### Triangulation

In our supervision of qualitative research studies, we emphasize the benefits of a triangulated approach to validity, which can include the literature review as one leg of the validity triangle (Hart, 2000). Triangulation as a strategy is based on the idea that different perspectives on the same phenomenon can enhance our understanding whilst at the same time can provide a basis for cross-checking and cross-referencing our findings. So triangulation is a strategy for enhancing validity, and validity approaches can themselves be triangulated at a meta level of analysis. For example, with the former, different methods of data analysis might be used to explore the same data set, or different perspectives might be elicited within the same data set (case study series with young women with a diagnosis of anorexia nervosa: their experience of living with the condition might be explored through a combination of in-depth interviewing with themselves, their carer(s) and their therapist; or their experience could be explored through in-depth interviews, psychometric measures and observation of a family mealtime). With the latter, the same study might use a number of approaches to the validity of the data analysis and the findings, such as a combination of respondent validation, face validity, independent audit and the clarity of the audit trail. These will be discussed in turn.

### Respondent validation

Respondent validation, sometimes called member validation or member checks, refers to those procedures whereby we take our findings back to our research participants and seek their views on our interpretations of the data. This process has the potential to increase the mutual understandings of the researcher and the research participants. Respondent validation is often used when the researcher is attempting to represent the views, opinions and experiences of the research participants, using such data analytic methods as IPA, theme analysis and grounded theory. Here, we want to try to get as close as possible to what people are saying, even though our understanding is filtered through our own 'perceptual lenses'.

The focus group format is one useful and time efficient way for feeding back our interpretation of the data. The focus group allows us to present our findings to either a selection of the original research participants or a representative group. To use our example above, it might be some of the young women with a diagnosis of anorexia nervosa who form our focus group, or another similar group of young women, so described. The value of a focus group for this purpose is that it can also represent another stage in the development of the research question. Thus, the very act of feeding back findings and inviting respondents' views takes the discussion on, for example, into applications of the findings, relevance for professional training, questions for further research, critique of the research question and so on. Ethically speaking, such an approach constitutes further intervention into people's lives and invites them to be thoughtful around their initial responses in ways not usually found in life.

## Concurrent/contextual validity

Concurrent or contextual validity is the extent to which the research relates to other work in the same field of enquiry. We often see concurrent validity explored and established through the literature review. The research question, as we frame it and ask it in a study, needs to be seen to arise naturally out of the literature review. A good literature review will help the reader of our research study to understand why this particular research question is being asked. The literature review will place the research question in the context of previous enquiry and clinical thinking and show how it will develop and advance understanding and practice. Thus our research question is shown to have validity. The validity of our research findings is also established with the help of the literature review. When we present and discuss our findings, we need to address the relationship between our research findings and their interpretation *and* our discussion of other related research and clinical thinking as presented in our literature review. Thus we discuss how our findings sit in the context of the work we reviewed in our literature review. The key validity question is: where are the similarities and differences, and how can we explain any discrepancies?

## The audit trail

The audit trail, the internal coherence of our findings and/or presentation of the evidence are terms used to describe the rhetorical power of the arguments the researcher puts forward in support of their findings and interpretation. For us as research supervisors, this is a core issue in establishing the validity and usefulness of our findings. A fine balance needs to be struck between an overly modest discussion of research findings, whereby their explanatory potential is not properly exploited, and an overly ambitious discussion of research findings, where cause–effect relationships are inferred or generalization is attempted beyond what the findings actually permit. Unsubstantiated claims to generalizability are a common problem we encounter in the writings of our research students. In our view, this can be forgiven at the first draft stage of writing because of enthusiasm and eagerness to lay claim to some findings of substance and because, we believe, ordinary English assumes cause–effect relationships in many idiomatic ways of speaking. The answer in our view comes in paying attention to detail. We encourage our students to re-read their own writing and examine every statement that makes a claim: can they support the claim with a well worked-out argument, or is it merely an assertion? If it is an assertion, we suggest they rewrite the claim using more tentative language, making clear that it is more a suggestion, prompted by their research experience, and is open to further investigation. We always suggest that the discussion of the research findings not only includes a critical appraisal of the research so conducted but also makes suggestions for further research, based on the findings.

The research findings need to have a degree of internal consistency and coherence. Clearly, if we use a strategy of triangulation within qualitative and mixed method enquiry, such as different perspectives on the same issue, we shall expect to find both differences and similarities in those perspectives (such as interviews with parents, adolescents and their therapists). If we use different methods of data collection, we will expect them to enrich our understanding of the issue at hand (such as observation, interviews and psychometric tests with adolescents). The key issue is how we theoretically integrate those differences and similarities, or use the differences to develop and challenge existing theory and clinical practice. Some differences in perspectives can be anticipated a priori. For example, research by the Beavers group on the development of self-report measures of family functioning, based in the Beavers model, predicted differences between adolescents' and parents' self-report and more similarity between adolescents' and outside observers' reports of family functioning. These predictions were born out in successive replications, supporting the Beavers model's theoretical prediction of adolescent differentiation. However, they were surprised to find that fathers' views correlated least with the outside observers, with mothers' views in an intermediate position between fathers' and adolescents' views. This gender difference in the parents' views prompted them to revise their model further in an effort to explain why fathers presented the most positive views of family functioning, relative to mothers, and to adolescents and outside observers (Beavers and Hampson, 1993).

The audit trail can be likened to showing our methods of calculation when doing long division or multiplication in our childhood arithmetic classes! We need to show the readers of our research how we moved from our raw data through the successive phases of our data analysis to reach our findings and their interpretation. If, for example, we are doing a discursive or grounded analysis of interview material, we need to show at each stage of our reading, and our analysis, how our findings are grounded in actual quotations from the interviews. Although discursive reading brings a higher level of inference to the interpretation of the data than do the grounded methods of analysis, the reader still needs to see and understand how the conclusions have been reached. When grounded methods are used, like theme analysis, IPA and grounded theory, a typical strategy is to include a selected sample of suitably anonymized pages from a sample of interview transcripts which show the original margin notes and codings, in an appendix. This supplements the presentation of the results, whereby each level of coding and categorization is shown in relation to the previous level and is supported at each stage by relevant direct quotations.

## Independent audit

Independent audit is the term used for those methods of establishing validity that most closely resemble the use of reliability in quantitative research. Independent audit checks for the transparency of the data analysis such that an independent reader can follow the analysis. When analysing interview transcripts, a typical approach is to recruit an independent reader who knows something of the topic being researched, giving them a sample of the data analyses, and asking them to read both the transcripts and the analyses to see if they can follow the analysis trail. Putting it simply, will the analysis make sense to them, given their own reading of the transcripts? A reliability study would be interested to compare the separate analyses of two independent analysts, whereas an independent audit is more interested to validate the coherence and relevance of an existing analysis. Once the independent auditor has read the transcripts and checked the data analysis, the auditor meets with the researcher to discuss how and where the data analysis makes sense to them and where they cannot follow it. In those instances, the two discuss their differences, with the researcher explaining why they analysed the data in the way they did, and the auditor explaining why it does not make sense to them. It is in the resolution of these differences that the original data analysis might be adjusted to accommodate the independent auditor's views.

## Self-reflexivity

There are other approaches to independent audit. A research diary or reflective journal is one method widely used. We favour keeping a reflective journal as the basis of the self-reflexive analysis required of researchers using qualitative methods. A reflective journal can be compiled during the whole of the research process, noting thoughts, emotional reactions, research decisions, theoretical linkings and connections with clinical practice, and comments on consultation and supervision to our research, both formal and informal. These varied jottings can be used to help us write retrospectively about our research journey, our motivation for doing the research, our personal biases as they were expressed and developed during the formulation of the research question and the collection and analysis of data. In particular, these jottings help us critically scrutinize our approach to data collection and analysis and pay attention to the influence and direction of our biases when writing the 'mea culpa' section of our discussion of our research findings. This critical analysis can be the golden thread of our approach to self-reflexivity throughout our research writing. A useful strategy is to subject the reflective journal to a theme analysis in its own right, to help tease out the different threads of our personal motivation, the influence of our clinical experience, our reliance on some theoretical ideas over others, our wish for positive outcomes and any tendency to underplay disconfirmatory instances in the data and in the findings.

When considering self-reflexivity, we find most researchers struggle at some level to articulate to others, let alone themselves, their own position in relation to the research question, the mode of enquiry and the data analysis and interpretation. A method we use to get the process started is to ask the researcher to invite a close colleague to interview them about their own reflexive position in relation to their research. The researcher and the chosen interviewer can collaborate to formulate the areas of enquiry for the interview, such as motivation, relevant personal and professional experience, areas of potential bias and so on. The colleague interviewer can then be relied upon to challenge and push the researcher's thinking, acting as a sounding board and giving feedback in response to the researcher. Thus the researcher's thinking about themselves in relation to their research enquiry can be articulated and developed. This interview could be repeated during and near the end of the research process. The interview should be audio-recorded and possibly, but not necessarily, transcribed. Similarly to the reflective journal, the self-reflexive interviews can be subjected to a theme analysis.

## Voice relational consultation

A further approach to independent audit and self-reflexivity that we wish to consider is voice relational consultation, first developed by Carol Gilligan (1982). This approach involves convening a small panel, say of three people, who will consult with the researcher about possible areas of bias and influence and how they think that might play out in the research process. Carol Gilligan, as a white, middle-class, articulate and older researcher, was interested to explore the experiences of young teenaged mothers, who were also black and living in poverty. Concerned that she and her colleagues might miss aspects of these young mothers' experiences, they convened a panel of research consultants to help them identify and understand their own sources of bias in relation to the material collected and analysed. The panel consisted of younger and older black women, with more or less formal educational experience.

Another example of the use of voice relational consultation can be found in Catherine Amor's (2000) grounded theory study of men's emotional well-being following vasectomy. As a woman who could not have a vasectomy she wondered what she might miss in the data. She convened a panel of three: her research supervisor (a woman); a male colleague who had not had a vasectomy; and a male colleague who had had a vasectomy. All three knew her well and were researchers themselves. They read samples of her interview transcripts with the male participants in her study and commented on what they 'saw' in the data, and what they thought she might be inclined to overplay and to underplay. Their written feedback to her was incorporated within her approach to analysis and within her critical review of her research.

## Generativity

The final approach to validity we wish to consider here is that of generativity, the extent to which the research findings can generalize to theory or population and have implications for clinical practice and training. As we have discussed in Chapter 3, qualitative research usually relies on small-scale approaches using theoretical or adventitious sampling in a 'local' study. The main aim of the research is usually to advance understanding within the context of the study sample. Thus any generalizability of the findings will be held within the potential for theory development or hypothesis generation around new lines of enquiry. Grounded theory methods have as their rationale the development of middle range theory, but other qualitative methods, such as IPA and the discursive and narrative methods of analysis, wish to make a contribution to theory development, although that might not be the main aim of the study. For us, the longer-term contribution of qualitative approaches to clinical research and their 'local' findings will lie in their social utility, that is, their collective contribution to a growing understanding and explanatory basis for clinical practice across settings, dilemmas and difference.

## CHAPTER SUMMARY

Throughout this book we encourage reflexivity in relation to our research activity and we see the importance of this not least in our approach to validity. Careful consideration of our values, motives and intentions allows us to reflect on how we influence the research process and how involvement in research impacts on us. We suggest a number of ways in which we can stay reflexive, such as regular consultation and supervision, keeping a research journal and taking part in self-reflexive research interviews. Collaborative research designs involve participants from the start, where possible. Building in approaches to validity that seek participants' views on the interpretation of the findings, or colleagues' views on the clinical and theoretical utility of the work, goes some way towards keeping the research grounded in experience. Asking participants and colleagues what they want from the research, or what they might get out of it, prepares the ground for the development of a do-able research design. All of this contributes to a style of working that reduces isolation and pays attention to issues of reciprocity from the start.

# FINAL REFLECTIONS

Research into psychotherapy can take a variety of forms and use a range of methods. In conducting research we have seen how we need to consider not only the very nature of psychotherapy but also the nature of psychological problems. How we define a problem determines what we think psychotherapy should be directed towards, and this in turn shapes how we set about attempting to do research. Central to this consideration is that our clients are often considered to be 'unusual', 'deviant', 'odd', 'bizarre' or 'pathological'. It is as if they fall outside what is deemed to be normal. In traditional research in the social sciences, however, much of the methods and statistical analyses have been based on ideas of normality as defined by the normal distribution. In fact, within this approach people who fall at the extremes have often been eliminated from studies on the basis that they are 'too extreme' and essentially 'mess up' the possible analysis, or are lost in a group averaging process. But in clinical work it is precisely the people who may be 'falling off the edge' of the distribution, the statistical 'outliers', so called, that we need to include. Hence in this book we have emphasized approaches, such as case studies and qualitative methods, that to us are more able to consider uniqueness and difference within local practice contexts. However, this is not to say that we wish to marginalize quantitative and statistical approaches, but rather that they have other uses and purposes.

A second important strand in our book has been that clients are people, with important ideas about what they want, what they need, and how to achieve this. Above all, this involves a recognition that in our research we are dealing with people who have understandings, intentions, hopes and fears. We question to what extent we include their views in our research aims and designs, either directly or indirectly. We have steered away from terms such as patients or subjects, and even have some reservation about the term 'client', though it does benefit from including a meaning of having intention and choice, even of seeking help rather than having treatment done to them or on them. In some aspects of counselling and psychotherapy, though, this assumption does not always hold. Some 'clients' do in fact experience considerable pressure, if not coercion and compulsion, to engage in treatment. We have seen, though, that this is a central issue in the efficacy of psychotherapy. How people come to engage in it shapes the relationship they can have with their therapist. It is the nature of this relationship that has consistently been found to be one of the central ingredients determining the efficacy of psychotherapy.

In this book we have described some of what we regard to be the substantial issues and methods in conducting research into psychotherapy. Broadly, we have suggested that this can be seen within three areas of activity:

- Research on the effectiveness of psychotherapy
- Research on the process of psychotherapy – how it works
- Research that furthers understanding of the underlying psychological and implicit theories that guide therapy.

These are interconnected activities. From the outset we have emphasized that any research inevitably is located within theories, though sometimes these are not made explicit. For example, when we decide that our measures will be participants' behaviours, this in itself makes a theoretical assumption that behaviour is the fundamental feature of therapeutic change rather than, say, beliefs or even more deeply concealed unconscious processes.

Above all, we have suggested that in psychotherapy research we need to think more broadly and critically about what we mean by research. Along with this, we need to think about why we might want to privilege this activity. In the chapter on case study research for example (Chapter 7), we have suggested that there is considerable overlap between a good clinical case report and a research case study:

- Careful consideration of our case or sample
- Respect for our participants and of ethical issues
- Detailed and comprehensive description of our case – history, context
- Systematic analysis and use of levels of analysis
- Reflective and critical analysis
- Careful consideration of data and evidence
- Use of data and evidence to support arguments and conclusions
- Development of local theory – grounded methods
- Use of self – careful analysis of our own role, assumptions and how these influence outcome
- Use of imagination and creativity
- Collaboration with our participant client in determining the goals, orientation, analysis and social utility of our research findings.

These pointers in fact apply to all forms of research into psychotherapy. We have suggested therefore that psychotherapy research needs to adopt a broad and flexible conceptualization of research. To emphasize this point, we can note that many of the most significant impacts on psychotherapy and clinical practice have come from studies that employ evocative descriptions, such as Freud's case studies, Goffman's vivid descriptions of an asylum and clients' reflections on their experiences in diary and journal studies. This is by no means an attempt to dismiss the relevance of quantitative evaluation studies. They have made an influential contribution to our evidence base and support our position of accountability around our practice. However, as we have suggested, it is important to complement these by accounts from the experiences of clients and therapists. Indeed, we might ask whether qualitative researchers have fudged this issue too. Clinicians and qualitative researchers might criticize the RCTs for over-generalizing their findings, and for limited applicability to working in the particular instance (with Mrs Smith!), but have qualitative researchers taken this seriously? Are we conducting too many local small-scale studies in isolation that cannot 'speak' to each other and collectively contribute to a broader base of knowledge?

How can these small-scale qualitative studies be combined with other small-scale studies to build up a body of knowledge? In our view, there are a number of potential ways forward. For example, adopting grounded theory methods of theoretical sampling will promote the development of shared, relevant knowledge about psychotherapy processes and outcomes. In addition, closer cooperation between psychotherapy and counselling training programmes will help advance much needed replication and further development of existing studies. There is a strong argument in our view for electronically networking student dissertations across course programmes to facilitate a more joined-up approach to small-scale qualitative and quantitative studies.

For us, the key points of importance are: using our clinical experience to help us set out on our research; to recognize and appreciate the complexity of our clinical thinking and practice and the wider definitions of research that flow from this; the importance of disseminating our small-scale study research findings more effectively (i.e. not leaving research dissertations to gather dust on library shelves); the wide variety in human experience that can only be captured with a willingness to use and recognize a wide variety of research designs; and the importance of effectiveness and efficacy research when considering the benefits or otherwise of our therapeutic approaches. Efficacy is defined as how much change treatments are seen to produce as opposed to how useful a treatment is in the heat of complex clinical practice.

In this book we have tried to show how psychotherapists and counsellors are uniquely positioned to do clinically relevant research. Their skills and wisdom, acquired and honed over years of practice, equip them in ways that they often do not recognize. Far from baulking at the suggestion of doing some applicable research, we would say 'go for it!' Psychotherapists and counsellors have acute powers of observation, the language for describing what they see in narrative and interactional detail and an understanding of how interviews work and of how to help people give their best in interviews. They also have a range of theoretical ideas that can drive analysis and/or complement a grounded analysis, an appreciation of ethical constraints and procedures, a capacity for attention to detail and to see the bigger picture and a wish to understand and explain, along with a clinically grounded appreciation of the importance of curiosity and scepticism. All of this experience and skill is immediately transferable into psychotherapy and counselling research activity.

We hope you have enjoyed reading this book and that it will encourage you in your research endeavours. Our imagination is engaged by doing research, just as it is when doing clinical work. When we can combine the best of clinical curiosity with research rigour we really feel connected to the people we work with, their concerns and priorities, in ways that take us further in our thinking, challenge some of our taken-for-granted assumptions and, most importantly of all, when supervising the work of students, make a contribution to the next generation of research activity.

# REFERENCES

Allport, G. W. (1962) *The Person in Psychology: Selected Essays*. Boston: Beacon Press.

American Psychiatric Association (1994) *Diagnostic and Statistical Manual of Mental Disorders*, 4th edn. Washington, DC: American Psychiatric Association.

Amor, C. (2000) *A Grounded Theory Approach to the Investigation of the Psychological Process of Vasectomy*. Unpublished Dissertation, Doctorate in Clinical Psychology, University of Surrey.

Andersen, T. (1987) The reflecting team: dialogue and meta-dialogue in clinical work, *Family Process*, 26: 415–28.

Arksey, H. (1996) Collecting data through joint interviews, *Social Research Update*, 15: 1–6.

Auburn, T. and Lea, S. (2003) Doing cognitive distortions: a discursive psychology analysis of sex offender treatment talk, *British Journal of Social Psychology*, 42: 281–98.

Bales, R. F. (1950) *Interaction Process Analysis: A Method for the Study of Small Groups*. Cambridge, MA: Addison-Wesley.

Bannister, D. and Fransella, F. (1971) *Inquiring Man*. London: Penguin.

Barker, C., Pistrang, N. and Elliott, R. (1994) *Research Methods in Clinical Psychology*. Chichester: Wiley.

Barker, C., Pistrang, N. and Elliott, R. (2002) *Research Methods in Clinical Psychology*, 2nd edn. Chichester: Wiley.

Barkham, M. (1989) Exploratory therapy in 2+1 sessions: I. Rationale for a brief psychotherapy model, *British Journal of Psychotherapy*, 6: 81–8.

Barlow, D. H. and Hersen, M. (1984) *Single Case Experimental Designs: Strategies for Studying Behaviour Change*. Oxford: Pergamon.

Barnard, C. P. and Kuehl, B. P. (1995) On-going evaluation: in-session procedures for enhancing the working alliance and therapy effectiveness, *The American Journal of Family Therapy*, 23(2): 161–72.

Bassey, M. (1998) Action research for improving educational practice, in R. Halsall (ed.) *Teacher Research and School Improvement: Opening doors from the inside*. Buckingham: Open University Press.

Bateson, G. (1972) *Steps to an Ecology of Mind*. New York: Ballantine.

Beavers, W. R. and Hampson, R. B. (1993) Measuring family competence: the Beavers Systems Model, in F. Walsh (ed.) *Normal Family Processes*, 2nd edn. New York: Guilford Press.

Beck, A. (1967) *Cognitive Therapy and Emotional Disorders*. New York: Harper & Row.

Beck, A. T., Rush, A. J., Shaw, B. F. and Emery, G. (1979) *Cognitive Therapy of Depression*. New York: Guilford Press.

Bem, D. (1994) Evaluating narrative family therapy: using single–system research designs, *Research on Social Work Practice*, 4(3): 309–25.

Benjamin, L. S. (1974) Structural analysis of social behaviour, *Psychological Review*, 81: 392–425.

Bennun, I. (1986) Evaluating family therapy: a comparison of the Milan and problem-solving approaches, *Journal of Family Therapy*, 8: 25–242.

Bennun, I., Chalkley, A. J. and Donnelly, M. (1987) Research applications of Shapiro's personal questionnaire in marital therapy, *Journal of Family Therapy*, 9: 131–44.

Ben Tovim, D. I. and Greenup, J. (1983) The representation of transference through serial grids. *British Journal of Medical Psychology*, 56: 255–62.

Bergin, A. (2003) *Bergin and Garfield's Handbook of Psychotherapy and Behavior Change*. New York: Wiley.

Blackburn, I. M. (1989) Severely depressed in-patient, in J. Scott, J. M. G. William and A. T. Beck (eds) *Cognitive Therapy in Clinical Practice*. London: Routledge.

Blatt, J. S., Sanislow III, C. A., Zuroff, D. C. and Pilkonins, P. A. (1996) Characteristics of effective therapists: further analysis from the National Institute of Mental Health Treatment of Depression and Collaborative Research Programme, *Journal of Consulting and Clinical Psychology*, 64(6): 1276–84.

Bolger, N., Davis, A. and Rafaeli, E. (2003) Diary methods: capturing life as it is lived, *Annual Review of Psychology*, 54: 579–616.

Bordin, E. (1979) The generalizability of the psychoanalytic concept of the working alliance, *Psychotherapy, Theory, Research and Practice*, 16: 252–60.

Borrill, J. and Foreman, E. I. (1996) Understanding cognitive change: a qualitative study of the impact of cognitive-behavioural therapy on fear of flying, *Clinical Psychology and Psycotherapy*, 3(1): 62–74.

Brown, G. W. and Harris, T. (1989) *The Social Origins of Depression*. London: Routledge.

Burbidge, C., Chamberlain, P. and Gallsworthy, L. (2004) Making outcomes measures work for psychologists, *Clinical Psychology*, 44, 30–33.

Burck, C. (2005) *Multi-lingual Living*. Basingstoke: Palgrave Macmillan.

Burman, E. and Parker, I. (1993) *Discourse Analytic Research: Repertoires and Readings of Texts in Action*. London: Routledge.

Burns, L. (2003) *An exploration of the place of literary reading in family therapists' personal and professional development*. Unpublished PhD thesis, University of Kent/Canterbury Christchurch University College.

Bussell, D. (1994) Ethical issues in observational family research, *Family Process*, 33: 361–76.

Bussell, D. A., Matsey, K. C., Reiss, D. and Hetherington, M. (1995) Debriefing the family: is research an intervention? *Family Process*, 34: 145–60.

Byng-Hall, J. (1995) Creating a secure base: some implications of attachment theory for family therapy, *Family Process*, 34: 45–58.

Casement, P. (1985) *Learning from the Patient*. London: Routledge.

Cecchin, G. (1987) Hypothesizing, circularity, and neutrality revisited: an invitation to curiosity, *Family Process*, 26(4): 405–13.

Charmaz, K. (1995) Grounded theory, in J. Smith, R. Harre and L. van Lagenhove (eds) *Rethinking Methods in Psychology*. London: Sage.

Cheseldine, S. (1995) Goal attainment scaling as an audit technique, *Clinical Psychology Forum*, 83: 18–22.

Clarke, C. and Llewelyn, S. (1994) Personal constructs of survivors of childhood sexual abuse receiving cognitive analytic therapy, *Journal of Medical Psychology*, 67: 273–89.

Cohen, J. (1988) *Statistical Power Analysis for the Behavioral Sciences*, 2nd edn. Hillsdale, NJ: Erlbaum.

Cook, T. D. and Campbell, D. T. (1979) *Quasi-experimentation: Design and Analysis for Field Settings*. Chicago: Rand-McNally.

Coulehan, R., Friedlander, M. L and Heatherington, L. (1988) Transforming narratives: a change event in constructivist family therapy, *Family Process*, 37: 17–33.

Crittenden, P. M. (1995) Attachment and psychopathology, in S. Goldberg, R. Muir and J. Kerr (eds) *Attachment Theory: Social, Developmental, and Clinical Perspectives*. Hillsdale, New Jersey: The Analytic Press.

Crouch, W. and Wright, J. (2004) A qualitative investigation into deliberate self-harm at an adolescent mental health unit, *Clinical Child Psychology and Psychiatry*, in press.

Curle, C. and Mitchell, A. (2004) Hand in hand: user and carer involvement in training clinical psychologists, *Clinical Psychology*, 33: 12–16.

Dalkey, N. (1972) *Studies in the Quality of Life*. Lexington, MA: Lexington Books.

Dallos, R. (2004) Attachment narrative therapy: integrating ideas from narrative and attachment theory in systemic family therapy with eating disorders, *Journal of Family Therapy*, 26(1): 40–66.

Dallos, R. and Draper, R. (2000) *An Introduction to Family Therapy*. Buckingham: Open University Press.

Dallos, R., Neale, A. and Strouthos, M. (1997) Pathways to problems: the evolution of 'pathology', *Journal of Family Therapy*, 19(4): 369–401.

Davey, G. (2003) What is interesting isn't always useful, *Psychologist*, 16(8): 412–16.

Derogatis, L. R., Lipman, R. S. and Covi, M. D. (1973) SCL-90, an outpatient rating scale: preliminary report, *Psychopharmacology Bulletin*, 9: 13–20.

Drummond, N. and Mason, C. (1990) Diabetes in a social context: just a different way of life in the age of reason, in S. Cunningham-Burley and N. P. McKeganey (eds) *Readings in Medical Sociology*. London: Routledge.

Duncan, B. and Miller, S. (2000) *The Heroic Client: Doing Client-directed Outcome Informed Therapy*. San Francisco: Jossey-Bass.

Elliott, R. (1984) A discovery-oriented approach to significant change events in psychotherapy: Interpersonal Process Recall and Comprehensive Process Analysis, in L. N. Rice and L. S. Greenberg (eds) *Patterns of Change: Intensive Analysis of Psychotherapy Process*. New York: Guilford Press.

Elliott, R. (1986) Interpersonal Process Recall (IPR) as a process research method, in L. Greenberg and W. Pinsof (eds) *The Psychotherapeutic Process*. New York: Guilford Press.

Elliott, R. (1989) Comprehensive process analysis: understanding the change process in significant events, in M. J. Packer and R. B. Addison (eds) *Entering the Circle: Hermeneutic Investigation in Psychology*. Albany, NY: SUNY Press.

Elliott, R. (1991) Five dimensions of therapy process, *Psychotherapy Research*, 1(2): 92–103.

Elliott, R., Fischer, C. T. and Rennie, D. L. (1999) Evolving guidelines for publication of qualitative research studies in psychology and related fields, *British Journal of Clinical Psychology*, 38: 215–29.

Elliot. R., Reminscuessel, C., Cislo, C. and James, E. (1984) *Therapeutic Impacts Content Analysis System*. Unpublished manuscript, University of Toledo.

Elliot, R. and Shapiro, D. A. (1988) Brief Structured Recall: a more efficient method for studying significant therapy events, *British Journal of Medical Psychology*, 61: 141–53.

Elliott, R., Shapiro, D. A., Firth-Cozens, J., Stiles, W. B., Hardy, G. E., Llewelyn, S. P. and Margison, F. R. (1994) Comprehensive Process Analysis of insight events in cognitive-behavioral and psychodynamic-interpersonal psychotherapies, *Journal of Counseling Psychology*, 41: 449–63.

Eysenck, H. J. (1952) The effects of psychotherapy, *Journal of Consulting and Clinical Psychology*, 16: 319–24.

Fairburn, C. G. and Brownell, K. D. (2002) *Eating Disorders and Obesity*. London: Guilford Press.

Falikov, C. (1998) *Latino Families in Therapy: A Guide to Multicultural Practice*. New York: Guilford Press.

Fern, E. (2001) *Advanced Focus Group Research*. London: Sage.

Festinger, L., Riecken, H. W. and Schacter, S. (1956) *When Prophecy Fails*. Minneapolis: University of Minnesota Press.

Fisher, R. A. (1935) *The Design of Experiments*. Edinburgh: Oliver and Boyd.

Flick, U. (2002) An Introduction to Qualitative Research, 2nd edn. London: Sage.

Fonagy, P., Steele, M., Steele, H., Higgit, A. and Target, M. (1994) The Emanuel Miller Memorial Lecture 1992, The theory and practice of resilience, *Journal of Child Psychiatry*, 35: 231–57.

Foucault, M. (1967) *Madness and Civilisation*. London: Tavistock.

Fraenkel, P. (1995) The nomothetic-idiograpic debate in family therapy, *Family Process*, 34: 113–121.

Freud, S. (1981) *Vol. 10. On Psychopathology*. Harmondsworth: Penguin.

Frosh, S., Burck, C., Strickland-Clark, L. and Morgan, K. (1996) Engaging with change: a process study of family therapy, *Journal of Family Therapy*, 18: 141–61.

Frosh, S., Phoenix, A. and Pattman, R. (2000) 'But it's racism I really hate': Young masculinities, racism, and psychoanalysis, *Psychoanalytic Psychology*, 17(2): 225–42.

Gale, J. (1992) When research interviews are more therapeutic than therapy interviews, *The Qualitative Report*, 1(4), 1–4.

Gergen, K. (1999 ) *An Invitation to Social Constructionism*. London: Sage.

Gilgun, J. F. (1994) A case for case studies in social work research, *Social Work*, 39: 370–80.

Gilgun, J. F. (1995) We shared something special: the moral discourse of incest perpetrators, *Journal of Marriage and the Family*, 57: 265–81.

Gill, R. (1996) Discourse analysis: practical implementation, in J. T. E. Richardson (ed.) *Handbook of Qualitative Research Methods for Psychology and the Social Sciences*. Leicester: BPS.

Gilligan, C. (1982) *In a Different Voice: Psychological Theory and Women's Development*. Cambridge, MA: Harvard University Press.

Glaser, B. G. and Strauss, A. L. (1967) *The Discovery of Grounded Theory: Strategies for Qualitative Research*. Chicago: Aldine.

Goffman, E. (1959) *The Presentation of Self in Everyday Life*. Garden City, NY: Doubleday-Anchor.

Goffman, E. (1961) *Asylums*. Chicago: Aldine.

Goldberg, D. (1992) GHQ-12: General Health Questionnaire. Windsor, UK: NFER-Nelson.

Goldberg, D. and Huxley, P. (1980) *Mental Illness in the Community: The Pathway to Psychiatric Care*. London: Tavistock.

Goldberg, D. and Huxley, P. (1992) *Common Mental Disorders*. London: Routledge.

Gomm, R., Hammersley, M. and Foster, P. (2000) Case study and generalization, in R. Gomm, M. Hammersley and P. Foster (eds) *Case Study Method*. London: Sage.

Greenberg, L. and Safran, J. (1987) *Emotion in Psychotherapy*. New York: Guilford Press.

Haley, J. (1987) *Problem Solving Therapy*, 2nd edn. San Fransisco: Jossey-Bass.

Hamlyn, D. W. (1970) *The Theory of Knowledge*. Garden City, NY: Doubleday-Anchor.

Hardy, G. E., Rees, A., Barkham, M., Field, S. D., Elliott, R. and Shapiro, D. A. (1998) Whingeing versus working: Comprehensive Process Analysis of a 'vague awareness' even in psychodynamic-interpersonal therapy, *Psythotherapy Research*, 8(3): 334–53.

Harre, R. and Secord, P. F. (1972) *The Explanation of Social Behaviour*. Oxford: Basil Blackwell.

Hart, C. (2000) *Doing a Literature Review: Releasing the Social Science Research Imagination*. London: Sage.

Harvey, J. H. Orbuch, T. L. and Weber, A. L. (eds) (1992) *Attributions, Accounts and Close Relationships*. London: Springer-Verlag.

Hayes, A. M., Goldfried, M. R. and Castonguay, L. G. (1996) The study of change in psychotherapy: a re-examination of the process-outcome correlation paradigm. Comment on Stiles and Shapiro (1994), *Journal of Consulting and Clinical Psychology*, 64: 909–14.

Heider, F. (1958) *The Psychology of Interpersonal Relations*. New York: Wiley.

Heller, T., Reynolds, J., Gomm, R., Muston, R. and Pattison, S. (1996) *Mental Health Matters*. London: Macmillan.

Helmeke, K. and Sprenkle, D. (2000) Clients' perceptions of pivotal moments in couples therapy: a qualitative study of change in therapy, *Journal of Marital and Family Therapy*, 26: 469–83.

Hilliard, R. B., Henry, W. P. and Strupp, H. H. (2000) An interpersonal model of psychotherapy: linking patient and therapist developmental history, therapeutic process and type of outcome, *Journal of Consulting and Clinical Psychology*, 68(1): 125–33.

Hollway, W. (1989) *Subjectivity and Method in Psychology: Gender, Meaning and Science*. London: Sage.

Hollway, W. and Jefferson, T. (2000) *Doing Qualitative Research Differently: Free Association, Narrative and the Interview Method*. London: Sage.

Hollway, W. and Jefferson, T. (2001) Free association, narrative analysis and the defended subject: The case of Ivy, *Narrative Inquiry*, 11(1): 103–22.

Honos-Webb, L., Stiles, W. B., Greenberg, L. S. and Goldman, R. (1998) Assimilation analysis of process-experiential psychotherapy: a comparison of two cases, *Psychotherapy Research*, 8(3): 264–86.

Horvath, A. and Symonds, B. (1991) Relations between working alliance and outcome in psychotherapy, *Journal of Counselling Psychology*, 38: 139–49.

Houston, J. (1998) *Making Sense with Offenders: Personal Construct Therapy and Change*. Chichester: Wiley.

Howard, K. I., Lueger, R. J., Maling, M. S. and Martinovich, Z. (1993) A phase model of psychotherapy outcome: causal mediation of change, *Journal of Consulting and Clinical Psychology*, 61(4): 678–85.

Jackson, D. (1957) The question of family homeostasis, *Psychiatry Quarterly Supplement*, 31: 79–99.

Jehu, D. (1988) *Beyond Sexual Abuse: Therapy with Women Who Were Victims in Childhood*. Chichester: Wiley.

Jones, E. (2003) Reflections under the lens: observations of a systemic therapist on the experience of participation and scrutiny in a research project, *Journal of Family Therapy*, 25(4): 347–57.

Jones, E. and Asen, E. (2000) *Systemic Couple Therapy and Depression*. London: Karnac.

Junker, B. H. (1972) *Fieldwork: An Introduction to the Social Sciences*. Chicago, Illinois: University of Chicago Press.

Kelly, G. A. (1955) *The Psychology of Personal Constructs*, Vols 1 and 2. New York: Norton.

Kirkman, M. (1999) Revising the plot: Autobiographical narratives after infertility. Available at http://www.latrobe.edu.au/aqr/offers/papers/MKirkman.htm

Kleinmann, A. (1988) *The Illness Narrative, Suffering, Healing and the Human Condition*. New York: Basic Books.

Kobak, R. and Cole, H. (1994) Attachment and meta-monitoring: implications for adolescent autonomy and psychopathology, in D. Cichetti and S. C. Toth (eds) *Disorders and Dysfunctions of the Self*. Based on papers presented at the 5th Annual

Rochester Symposium on Developmental Psychopathology, vol. 5, University of Rochester Press: Rochester, New York.

Krause, L. B. (1995) Personhood, culture and family therapy, *Journal of Family Therapy*, 17(4): 363–82.

Kuhn, T. (1970) *The Structure of Scientific Revolutions*. Chicago: University of Chicago Press.

Labov, W. and Fanshel, D. (1977) *Therapeutic Discourse*. New York: Academic Press.

Laing, R. D. and Esterson, A. (1964) *Sanity, Madness and the Family*. London: Tavistock.

Lamiel, J. T. (1998) 'Nomothetic' and 'Idiographic': contrasting Windlebands' understanding with contemporary usage, *Theory and Psychology*, 8(10): 23–38.

Landfield, A. W. (1971) *Personal Construct Systems in Psychotherapy*. Lincoln: University of Nebraska.

Lask, J. and Vetere, A. (2003) Editorial. *Journal of Family Therapy*, 25(4): 315–16.

Leff, J. and Vaughn, C. (1985) *Expressed Emotions in Families: Its Significance for Mental Illness*, New York, Guilford Press.

Leff, J., Vearnals, S. Brevin, C. R., Wolff, G., Alexander, B., Asen, K., Dayson, D., Jones, E., Chisholm, D. and Everitt, B. (2000) The London Depression Intervention Trial. Randomised control trial of antidepressants vs couple therapy in the treatment and maintenance of people with depression living with a critical partner: clinical outcome and costs, *British Journal of Psychiatry*, 177: 95–100.

Leiper, R. (2001) *Working Through Setbacks in Psychotherapy*. London: Sage.

Linstone, H. and Turoff, M. (eds) (1975) *The Delphi Method: Techniques and Applications*. Reading, MA: Addison Wesley Publishers.

Littlewood, R. and Lipsedge, M. (1982) *Aliens and Alienists: Ethnic Minorities and Psychiatry*. Harmondsworth: Penguin.

Llewelyn, S. P., Elliot, R., Shapiro, D. A., Hardy, G. and Firth-Cozens, J. (1988) Client perceptions of significant events in prescriptive and exploratory periods of individual therapy, *British Journal of Clinical Psychology*, 27: 105–14.

Lobatto, W. (2002) Talking to children about family therapy: a qualitative research study, *Journal of Family Therapy*, 24(3): 330–43.

London, I. D. and Thorngate, W. (1981) Divergent amplification and social behaviour: some methodological considerations, *Psychological Reports*, 48: 203–28.

Luborsky, L., Critis-Cristoph, P., Leslie-Alexander, M. S., Margolis, M. and Cohen, M. (1983) Two helping alliance methods for predicting outcome of psychotherapy, *Journal of Nervous and Mental Disease*, 171(8): 480–91.

Maclachlan, A. and Newnes, C. (2002) The information, *Clinical Psychology*, 16: 12–15.

Mason, B. (2003) *The Development of a Relational Approach to the Understanding, Treatment and Management of Chronic Pain*. Unpublished Doctoral Thesis, University of East London/Tavistock Centre.

Mason, B. (2004) A relational approach to the management of chronic pain, *Clinical Psychology*, 35: 17–20.

Mason, J. (2002) *Qualitative Researching*, (2nd edn). London: Sage.

Maxwell, J. (1996) *Qualitative Research Design: An Interactive Approach*. Thousand Oaks, CA: Sage.

Meehl, P. (1978) Theoretical risks and tabular asterisks: Sir Karl, Sir Ronald, and the slow progress of soft psychology, *Journal of Consulting and Clinical Psychology*, 46: 806–834.

Minuchin, S., Rosman, B. L. and Baker, L. (1978) *Psychosomatic Families: Anorexia Nervosa in Context*. Cambridge, MA: Harvard University Press.

Morley, S. and Adams, M. (1989) Some simple statistical tests for exploring single-case time-series data, *British Journal of Clinical Psychology*, 28: 1–18.

Mullender, A., Hague, G., Imam, U., Kelly, L., Malos, E. and Regan, L. (2002) *Children's Perspectives on Domestic Violence*. London: Sage.

Neuendorf, K. A. (2002) *The Content Analysis Guidebook*. London: Sage.

Orne, M. T. (1962) On the social psychology of the psychological experiment with particular reference to demand characteristics and their implications, *American Psychologist*, 17: 776–83.

Osborn, M. and Smith, J. A. (1998) The personal experience of chronic benign lower back pain: an interpretative phenomenological analysis, *British Journal of Health Psychology*, 3: 65–83.

Pahl, J. (1989) *Money and Marriage*. Basingstoke: Macmillan.

Palazzoli, M. S. (1974) *Self-Starvation: From the Intrapsychic to the Transpersonal Approach to Anorexia Nervosa*. London: Human Context Books.

Parry, G. (2001) Introduction: Treatment choice in psychological therapies, *Evidence Based Clinical Practice Guidelines*. Department of Health, UK.

Parry, G., Shapiro, D. A. and Firth, J. (1986) The case of the anxious executive: a study from the research clinic, *British Journal of Medical Psychology*, 86: 221–33.

Patterson, G. R. and Forgatch, M. S. (1985) Therapist behaviour as a determinant for client non-compliance: a paradox for the behaviour modifier, *Journal of Consulting and Clinical Psychology*, 53(6): 846–51.

Pinsof, W. M. and Catherall, D. R. (1986) The integrative psychotherapy alliance: family, couple and individual therapy scales, *Journal of Marital and Family Therapy*, 12: 132–51.

Pinsof, W. M. and Wynne, L. C. (1995) The efficacy of marital and family therapy: an empirical overview, conclusions and recommendations, *Journal of Marital and Family Therapy*, 21: 585–613.

Pinsof, W. M. and Wynne, L. C. (2000) Toward progress research: closing the gap between family therapy practice and research, *Journal of Marital and Family Therapy*, 26(1): 1–8.

Popper, K. R. (1959) *The Logic of Scientific Discovery*. New York: Basic Books. (Original German edition 1934.)

Prochaska, J. O. and DiClemente, C. C. (1982) Transtheoretical therapy: toward a more integrative model of change, *Psychotherapy, Theory, Research and Practice*, 20: 161–73.

Prochaska, J. O., DiClemente, C. C. and Norcross, J. C. (1992) In search of how people change, *American Psychologist*, September: 1102–4.

Reid, K., Flowers, P. and Larkin, M. (2005) Exploring lived experience, *The Psychologist*, 18(1): 20–6.

Reimers, S. and Treacher, A. (1995) *Introducing User-Friendly Family Therapy*. London: Routledge.

Rennie, D. (1992) Qualitative analysis of client's experience of the psychotherapy: the unfolding of reflexivity, in S. G. Toukmanian and D. Rennie (eds) *Psychotherapy Process Research: Paradigmatic and Narrative Approaches*. London: Sage.

Riessman, C. K. (1993) *Narrative Analysis*. Newbury Park, CA: Sage.

Robinson, D. N. (2000) Paradigms and the myth of framework, *Theory and Psychology*, 10(1): 39–47.

Robson, C. (2002) *Real World Research*, 2nd edn. Oxford: Blackwell.

Rodriguez, N. and Ryave, A. (2002) *Systematic Self-Observation*. London: Sage.

Rogers, C. (1951) *Client Centred Therapy*. Boston: Houghton Mifflin.

Rogers, C. R. and Truax, C. B. (1965) The therapeutic conditions antecedent to change: a theoretical view, in L. Wynne (ed.) *The Therapeutic Relationship and its Impact: A Study of Psychotherapy with Schizophrenics*. Wisconsin: University of Wisconsin Press.

Rosenberg, M. (1965) *Society and Adolescent Self-image*. Princetown, NJ: Princetown University Press.

Rosenhan, D. L. (1973) Being sane in insane places, *Science*, 179, 250–8.

Rosenthal, R. (1976) *Experimental Effects in Behavioral Research*, rev. edn. New York: Irvington.

Roth, A. and Fonagy, P. (1996) *What Works for Whom? A Critical Review of Psychotherapy Research*. London: Guilford.

Rustin, M. (2002) Research, evidence and psychotherapy, in C. Mace, S. Morley and B. Roberts (eds) *Evidence in the Psychological Therapies*. Hove: Brunner-Routledge.

Ryle, A. (1990) *Cognitive-analytic Therapy: Active Participation in Change: A New Integration in Brief Therapy*. Chichester: Wiley.

Sacks, O. (1985) *The Man Who Mistook His Wife for a Hat*. London: Touchstone Books.

Safran, J. D., Crocker, P., McMain, S. and Murray, P. (1990) Therapeutic alliance ruptures as a therapy event for empirical investigation, *Psychotherapy*, 27(3): 154–65.

Salkovskis, P. (1989) Obsessions and compulsions, in J. Scott, J. M. G. Williams and A. T. Beck (eds) *Cognitive Therapy in Clinical Practice*. London: Routledge.

Salmon, P. (2003) How do we recognise good research? *The Psychologist*, 16(1): 24–7.

Sandberg, J. G., Johnson, L. N., Robila, M. and Miller, R. B. (2002) Clinician identified barriers to clinical research, *Journal of Marital and Family Therapy*, 28(1): 61–7.

Seale, C. (1999) *The Quality of Qualitative Research*. London: Sage.

Seltzer, M. and Seltzer, W. (2004) Co-texting, chronotope and ritual: a Bakhtinian framing of talk in therapy, *Journal of Family Therapy*, 26: 358–83.

Shapiro, D. A. (1975) Some implications of psychotherapy research for clinical psychology, *British Journal of Medical Psychology*, 48: 199–206.

Sixsmith, J. (2004) Young men's health and group participation: participatory research gone wrong? *Clinical Psychology*, 43: 13–18.

Skinner, B. F. (1953) *Science and Human Behaviour*. New York: Macmillan.

Sloane, R. B., Staples, F. R., Cristol, A. H., Yorkston, N. J. and Whipple, K. (1975) *Psychotherapy Versus Behavior Therapy*. Cambridge, MA: Harvard University Press.

Sluzki, C. E. (1992) Transformations: a blueprint for narrative changes in therapy, *Family Process*, 31: 217–30.

Sluzki, C. E. and Ransom, D. C. (eds) (1976) *Double Bind: The Foundations of the Communicational Approach to the Family*. New York: Grune and Stratton.

Smith, J. A. (1996) Beyond the divide between cognition and discourse: using interpretative phenomenological analysis in health psychology, *Psychology and Health*, 11: 261–71.

Smith, J. A., Osborn, M. and Jarman, M. (1999) Doing interpretative phenomenological analysis, in M. Murray and K. Chamberlain (eds) *Qualitative Health Psychology*. London: Sage.

Snelling, E. (2003) *Megan's story: Transitional Space and Places: Making Meaning of Turning Points in the Life of a Member of a Hearing Voices Group*. Unpublished Dissertation, Doctorate in Clinical Psychology, University of Plymouth.

Stancombe, J. and White, S. (1997) Notes on the tenacity of therapeutic presuppositions in process research: examining the artfulness of blamings in family therapy, *Journal of Family Therapy*, 19: 21–41.

Stapp, H. (1971) S-matrix interpretation of quantum theory, *Physical Review*, D3: 1303–20.

Stenner, P. (1993) Discoursing jealousy, in E. Burman and I. Parker (eds) *Discourse Analytic Research*. London: Routledge.

Stiles, W. B., Elliot, R., Llewelyn, S. P., Firth-Cozens, J. A., Margison. F. R., Shapiro, D. A. and Hardy, G. (1990) The assimilation of problematic experiences by clients in psychotherapy, *Psychotherapy*, 27(3): 411–20.

Stiles, W. B., Meshot, C. M., Anderson, T. T. and Sloan, W. W. (1992) Assimilation of problematic experiences: the case of John Jones, *Psychotherapy Research*, 2(2): 81–101.

Stiles, W. B., Shapiro, D. A. and Elliott, R. (1986) Are all psychotherapies equal, *American Psychologist*, 41(2): 165–80.

Stiles, W. B. and Shapiro, D. A. (1994) Abuse of the drug metaphor in psychotherapy process – outcome research, *Clinical Psychology Review*, 9: 521–43.

Stith, S. M., Rosen, K. H., McCollum, E. E., Coleman, J. U. and Herman, S. A. (1996) The voices of children: preadolescent children's experiences in family therapy, *Journal of Marital and Family Therapy*, 22: 69–86.

Stockwell, T., Murphy, D. and Hodgson, R. (1983). The severity of alcohol dependence questionnaire: its use, reliability and validity, *British Journal of Addiction*, 78: 145–55.

Stone Fish, L. and Busby, D. M. (1996) The Delphi Method, in D. H. Sprenkle and S. M. Moon (eds) *Research Methods in Family Therapy*. New York: Guilford Press.

Strauss, A. and Corbin, J. (1998) *Basics of Qualitative Research: Techniques and Procedures for Developing Grounded Theory*, 2nd edn. Newbury Park, CA: Sage.

Strickland-Clark, L., Campbell, D. and Dallos, R. (2000) Children's and adolescents' views on family therapy, *Journal of Marital Therapy*, 22(3): 324–41.

Strupp, H. H. (1986) The non-specific hypothesis of therapeutic effectiveness: a current assessment, *American Orthopsychiatric Association*, 56(4): 513–29.

Toukmanian, S. G. and Rennie, D. L. (eds) (1992) *Psychotherapy Process Research*. London: Sage.

Truax, C. B. (1966) Reinforcement and non-reinforcement in Rogerian Psychotherapy, *Journal of Abnormal Psychology*, 71(1): 1–9.

Turner, W. L. (2000) Cultural considerations in family-based primary prevention programs in drug abuse, *Journal of Primary Prevention*, 21(2): 285–303.

Van Roosmalen, M. (2001) *Therapist Intervention Factors that Influence Therapeutic Alliance Events in Family Therapy with Multi-problem Families: A Qualitative Study.* Unpublished Dissertation, Doctorate in Clinical Psychology, Canterbury, Christ Church University College.

Vetere, A. and Dallos, R. (2003) *Working Systemically with Families: Formulation, Intervention and Evaluation*. London: Karnac.

Vetere, A. and Gale, T. (1987) *Ecological Studies of Family Life*. Chichester: Wiley.

Vetere, A. and Myers, L. (2004) Families, coping styles and physical health, in R. Crane and E. Marshall (eds) *Handbook of Families and Health*. Thousand Oaks, CA: Sage.

Viljoen, D. and Wolpert, M. (2002) Increasing return rates from postal outcome questionnaires: ten pointers from the literature, *Clinical Psychology*, 19: 18–21.

Vostanis, P., Burnham, J. and Harris, Q. (1992) Changes of expressed emotion in systemic family therapy, *Journal of Family Therapy*, 14(1): 15–27.

Watzlawick, P. (1964) *An Anthology of Human Communication*. Palo Alto, CA: Science and Behaviour Books.

Watzlawick, P., Beavin, J. and Jackson, D. (1967) *Pragmatics of Human Communication*. New York: Norton.

Watzlawick, P., Weakland, J. and Fisch, R. (1974) *Change: Principles of Problem Formation and Problem Resolution*. New York: Norton.

Wessley, S. (2001) Randomised control trials, in C. Mace, S. Morley and B. Roberts (eds) *Evidence in the Psychological Therapies*. Hove: Brunner-Routledge.

Wetherell, M., Taylor, S. and Yates, S. (eds) (2001) *Discourse as Data: A Guide for Analysis*. London: Sage.

White, M. B. and Russell, C. S. (1995) The essential elements of supervisory systems: a modified Delphi study, *Journal of Marital and Family Therapy*, 21(1): 33–53.

Whyte, W. F. (1955) *Street Corner Society: The Social Structure of an Italian Slum*. Chicago, Illinois: University of Chicago Press.

Wicks, R. P. (1982) Interviewing: practical aspects, in A. J. Chapman and A. Gale (eds) *Psychology and People: A Tutorial Text*. Leicester: British Psychological Society and The Macmillan Press Ltd.

Williams, M. (2000) *Science and Social Science: An Introduction*. London: Routledge.

Wilson, B. (1987) Single case experimental designs in neuropsychological rehabilitation, *Journal of Clinical and Experimental Neuropsychology*, 9: 527–44.

Wing, J. K., Beevor, A. S., Curtis, R. H., Park, S. B., Hadden, S. and Burns, A. (1998).
Health of the Nation Outcome Scales: Research and development, *British Journal of
Psychiatry*, 172: 11–18.

Windleband, W. (1921) *An Introduction to Philosophy*. London: Unwin.

Winter, D. (2003) Repertory Grid Technique as a psychotherapy research measure,
*Psychotherapy Research*, 13(1): 25–42.

Wolcott, H.F. (1990) *Writing Up Qualitative Research*. London: Sage.

Wollheim, R. (1971) *Freud: Biologist of the Mind*. London: Fontana.

Woodward, C. and Joseph, S. (2003) Positive change processes and post-traumatic
growth in people who have experienced childhood abuse: understanding vehicles
of change, *Psychology and Psychotherapy-Theory Research and Practice*, 76: 267–83.

Woskett, K. (1999) *The Therapeutic Use of Self*. Hove: Brunner-Routledge.

Wynne, L. (1988) *The State of the Art in Family Therapy Research*. New York: Family
Process Press.

Yin, R. K. (1994) *Case Study Research: Design and Methods*, 2nd edn. Thousand Oaks,
CA: Sage.

# INDEX

neurological disorders, 129
Newnes, C., 87
nomothetic approach, 25–7, 34, 132
non-compliance, 120–2
non-verbal communication, 74, 179,
    180–1, 192–3
'normality', 7

objectivity, 9–10
observation, 52, 71–2, 74, 83, 102,
    160–75
  access to research participants, 169–71
  analysis of data, 162–3
  approaches to validity, 203–5
  centrality as a research tool, 161–2
  focus groups, 186–7
  interpretative observational analysis,
    160–1, 162–74, 181
  participant observation and depth
    interviewing, 194–9
  relationship to interviewing, 192–4
  social roles of participant observer,
    166–9
  special problems of participant
    observation, 171–4
  structured, 163, 174–5
observer as participant, 166–7, 168
obsessions, 140–1
ontology, 27
operant conditioning, 141–2
opportunistic sampling approach, 29,
    36
order, chronological, 69
Osborn, M., 57–8
outcome studies see evaluation and
    outcome
outliers, statistical, 36–7, 80, 211
own organizations, research within,
    173–4
own practice, research into, 103

Pahl, J., 184
pain, 57–8
Palazzoli, M.S., 164
paradigm shifts, 12
parent training, 121–2
Parker, I., 67
Parry, G., 11, 155, 156
participant observation, 71–2, 166–74
  access to research participants,
    169–71
  and depth interviewing, 194–9
  social roles of participant observer,
    166–9
  special problems of, 171–4

participant as observer, 166–7, 168
participants, research, 12
  access to, 169–71, 178, 197
  availability and motivation, 37–8
  and collaborative research see
    collaborative research
  selection of, 7–8
Pasteur, Louis, 7
pathological pathways, 68
pathways to mental health problems, 6
Patterson, G.R., 120–2
Pattman, R., 63
permission, 178
personal construct theory (PCT) case
    studies, 133, 148–55
personal experience narratives, 69
personal questionnaires, 133, 154–8
personality disorders, 6, 19–20
phases of psychotherapy, 89
phenomenology, 51
Phoenix, A., 63
physical disorders and conditions, 6
physiological change, 98
Pilkonis, P.A., 120
piloting, 18
  interviewing, 179, 186, 194–5
Pinsof, W.M., 82
pivotal moments, 54–5, 70
    see also significant events research
placebo treatments, 79, 96
pluralism, 83
political agendas, 19–20
Popper, K.R., 16
positivist epistemology, 27–8
post-traumatic growth, 62
power, 10
  and discursive approaches, 67
practice based evidence, 4–5, 81–3,
    141
pragmatic theory, 28
pre-contemplation, 124, 125–6
preliminary work, 18
probability sampling, 36
problem solving family therapy, 86
process of an interview, 180–1
process research see psychotherapy
    process research
Prochaska, J.O., 124–6
professionals, abuse by, 99
prototypical cases, 42
psychodynamic analysis, 64
psychodynamic approaches, 7
psychotherapy
  defining, 5–6
  meaning and experience of, 3–4

# AN INTRODUCTION TO FAMILY THERAPY
## SYSTEMIC THEORY AND PRACTICE
## SECOND EDITION

### Rudi Dallos and Ros Draper
*University of Plymouth; Institute of Family Therapy, UK*

This popular introduction to the theory and practice of family therapy offers a comprehensive overview of the core concepts and ideas that have developed in systemic theory from the 1950s to the present day. Thoroughly updated with the latest research and developments, and illustrated throughout with lively examples drawn from clinical practice, this user-friendly guide provides practical resources and suggestions for improved therapeutic practice.

New to this edition:

- A new chapter on systemic formulation
- A new chapter on practice development 2000–2004
- Increased coverage of the evidence base for the effectiveness of family therapy
- Stronger focus on attachment and psychodynamic perspectives
- Comprehensive references to key people, events and texts

Written by experienced authors, this essential resource is key reading for students and practitioners of family therapy as well as those from the fields of counselling, psychology, social work and the helping professions who deal with family issues.

*Contents*
*Preface – Introduction – The first phase – 1950s to mid-70s – The second phase – mid-1970s to mid-1980s – The third phase – mid-1980s–2000 – Ideas that keep knocking on the door – Systemic formulation – Current practice development 2000–2004 – Research and evaluation – Reflections and critique – Postscripts – Appendices – Index.*

360pp     0 335 21604 8 Paperback £24.99     0 335 21605 6 Hardback £60.00

# THE POLITICS OF PSYCHOTHERAPY
## NEW PERSPECTIVES

### Nick Totton (ed)
*Psychotherapist and trainer in private practice, UK*

A unique collection by leading authors, *The Politics of Psychotherapy* explores the links between therapy and the political world, and their contribution to each other. Topics covered include:

- Psychotherapy in the political sphere, including the roots of conflict, social trauma, and ecopsychology
- Political dimensions of psychotherapy practice, discrimination, power, sexuality, and postcolonial issues
- Psychotherapy, the state and institutions, including the law and ethics, and psychotherapy in healthcare
- Working at the Interface, examples of therapy in political action from Croatia, the USA, the UK and Israel/Palestine.

How to 'place' political issues in therapy is highly controversial – for example, whether political themes should be interpreted psychologically in the consulting room, or respected as valid in their own right: Similar issues arise for the role of therapeutic insights in political reality. This book provides a map through these complex and demanding areas for therapists and counsellors in training, and also for experienced practitioners and other interested readers.

### Contributors
*Lane Arye, Arlene Audergon, Emanuel Berman, Sandra Bloom, Jocelyn Chaplin, Petruska Clarkson, Chess Denman, Dawn Freshwater, Kate Gentile, Susan Gutwill, John Lees, Hilary Prentice, Mary-Jayne Rust, Judy Ryde; Andrew Samuels, Nick Totton.*

### Contents
*Acknowledgements – Notes on contributors – Introduction – Part 1: Psychotherapy in the political sphere – Politics on the couch? psychotherapy and society – some possibilities and some limitations – Societal trauma: democracy in danger – Conflict, competition and aggression – The breast-milk of the Inuit mother: a tale of micro and macrocosm, shadow and light – Part 2: Political dimensions of psychotherapy practice - The politics of sexuality, gender and object choice in therapy – Working with difference: the political context of psychotherapy with an intersubjective dialogue – Power in the therapeutic relationship – Part 3: Psychotherapy, the state and institutions – Values, ethics and the law: a story with some morals – The institutions of psychotherapy – Politics and psychotherapy in the context of healthcare – Part 4: Working at the interface: psychotherapy in political action – ransforming conflict into community: post-war reconciliation in croatia – Israeli psychotherapists and the Israeli-Palestinian conflict – The Bridge Project: radical psychotherapy for the 21st century – How to create social activism: turning the passive to active without killing each other – Index.*

192pp     0 335 21653 6 Paperback £19.99     0 335 21654 4 Hardback £60.00

# COUNSELLING SKILL

## John McLeod
*University of Abertay, Dundee, UK*

The sites or opportunities for counselling within our society include both formal counselling, usually provided by trained counsellors, psychotherapists and other mental health workers over a number of meetings, and informal episodes of counselling, provided by nurses, doctors, social workers, advice workers, teachers and other human service professionals. The provision of counselling by this latter group is typically described in terms of the use of "counselling skills", to differentiate it from formal, contracted, long-term counselling. Counselling skills interventions are usually delivered in the context of single episodes. This book is aimed at giving counselling skill to those who require a level of counselling for their chosen profession.

The idea of counselling skill (as opposed to skills) reflects a new way of conceptualising this kind of work. This conceptual model is explained in the introduction, and operates as a framework for the book as a whole. The model is derived from two basic ideas: Firstly, it is assumed that most people are able to do the things that are necessary in order to offer an effective counselling relationship: listen carefully, be reliable and trustworthy, be aware of feelings, check things out, etc. These are not special skills – they are everyday human attributes. What is skilful, it is argued, is an ability to bring these competencies together for a specific purpose. Secondly, the person seeking help is assumed to be an active agent who is attempting to use whatever resources are at his/her disposal in order to deal with the difficulties which he/she is confronted. From this perspective, the task of the counsellor or helper is not to offer solutions to the person's problem, but to create an arena within which they can work together to make use of whatever resources are available.

Topics covered include:

- A definition of counselling and exploration of counselling models and contexts
- Issues to consider in preparation for undertaking a counselling relationship
- Trust
- Confidentiality
- Listening and responding
- How to combine counselling with a professional role

The book features summary boxes and a running case study throughout, to illustrate the key themes. It is essential reading for those who use counselling in their professional work in social and allied health services.

### Contents
*Introduction – Preparation – Making a Space – Being there: listening, paying attention, witnessing – Responding to the other: facilitating learning and change – Putting it all together – Dealing with difficult situations – Doing good work – References – Index.*

224pp    0 335 21809 1 Paperback £19.99    0 335 21810 5 Hardback £60.00

# COUNSELLING SKILLS IN SOCIAL WORK PRACTICE
## SECOND EDITION

### Janet Seden
*The Open University, UK*

- In what ways is counselling relevant to contemporary social work?
- How do counselling skills integrate with social work roles and responsibilities?

This book examines these skills and their applicability, drawing from social work and counselling theories and methods using clear, practical examples. Skills are discussed with reference to social work knowledge and values illustrating how, when used competently, contextually and sensitively they can appropriately underpin good social work practice. Questions and activities for self development are linked to the practices discussed.

This new edition of *Counselling Skills in Social Work Practice* has been thoroughly revised to reflect the National Occupational Standards for social work which identify the importance of communication skills and a developmental understanding of people in their social contexts. The chapters are linked to the six key roles for social work practice.

This book builds on the strengths of the first edition, as well as addressing the challenges of practice in relevant legislative and policy contexts. The book includes:

- Evidence of how the competencies which underpin counselling practice are directly transferable to effective social work practice
- Practical advice on communication skills
- Examples of how to build effective working relationships; a whole chapter is now devoted to the specific skills required for working within inter-agency and multi-disciplinary teams

This book is key reading on the subject of ethical and effective social work for those teaching, studying or practising in the field.

### Contents
*Preface – Counselling skills and social work: a relationship – Counselling skills for communication – Assessing: relevant counselling skills – Planning, acting and providing a service: relevant counselling skills – Supporting service user choice and advocacy: relevant counselling skills – Managing risk and working together: relevant counselling skills – Practice within organizations: relevant counselling skills – Developing professional competence: relevant counselling skills – References – Index.*

192pp     0 335 21649 8 (Paperback)

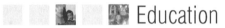
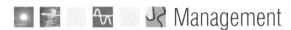
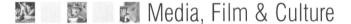
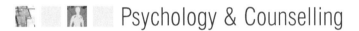
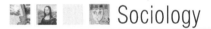
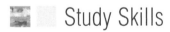
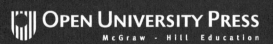
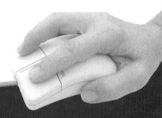